RADIOLOGY
POCKET REFERENCE

What To Order When

D0915759

RADIOLOGY
POCKET REFERENCE

What To Order When

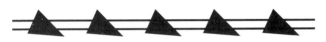

Ronald L. Eisenberg, MD
Clinical Professor of Radiology
University of California at San Francisco
University of California at Davis

Chairman of Radiology
Alameda County Medical Center
Oakland, California

Alexander R. Margulis, MD, DSc (hon)
Professor of Radiology
University of California at San Francisco

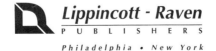

Lippincott - Raven
PUBLISHERS
Philadelphia • New York

Acquisitions Editor: James D. Ryan
Sponsoring Editor: Susan R. Skand
Production Editor: Sharon McCarthy
Production Manager: Janet Greenwood

Library of Congress Cataloging in Publication Data

Radiology pocket reference : what to order when / editors,
    Ronald L. Eisenberg and Alexander R. Margulis.
        p.   cm.
    Includes bibliographical references and index.
    ISBN 0-397-51503-0
    1. Diagnostic imaging—Handbooks, manuals, etc.
    I. Eisenberg, Ronald L.   II. Margulis, Alexander R.
    [DNLM: 1. Radiography—handbooks. WN 39 R1295 1996]
    RC78.7.D53R35   1996
    616.07′54—dc20
    DNLM/DLC
    for Library of Congress   96-11509
                                                                    CIP

The material contained in this volume was submitted as previously
unpublished material, except in the instances in which credit has
been given to the source from which some of the illustrative material was derived.

Great care has been taken to maintain the accuracy of the information contained in the volume. However, neither Lippincott–
Raven Publishers nor the editors can be held responsible for errors
or for any consequences arising from the use of the information
herein.

The authors and publisher have exerted every effort to ensure
that drug selection and dosage set forth in this text are in accord
with current recommendations and practice at the time of publication. However, in view of ongoing research, changes in government
regulations, and the constant flow of information relating to drug
therapy and drug reactions, the reader is urged to check the pack-
age insert for each drug for any change in indications and dosage
and for added warnings and precautions. This is particularly important when the recommended agent is a new or infrequently employed drug.

Materials appearing in this book prepared by individuals as part
of their official duties as U.S. Government employees are not cov-
ered by the above-mentioned copyright.

9   8   7   6   5   4   3   2   1

To Zina, Avlana, and Cherina
and
To Hedi

Contributors

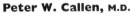

Peter W. Callen, M.D.
Professor of Radiology,
    Obstetrics, Gynecology
    and Reproductive Science
University of California
    School of Medicine
San Francisco, California

William Dillon, M.D.
Professor of Radiology,
    Neurology and
    Neurosurgery
Chief of Neuroradiology
University of California
    School of Medicine
San Francisco, California

**Burton P. Drayer,
M.D.**
Chairman, Department of
    Radiological Sciences
Director of Magnetic
    Resonance Imaging
St. Joseph's Hospital and
    Medical Center
Barrow Neurological Institute
Phoenix, Arizona

N. Reed Dunnick, M.D.
Professor and Chair
Department of Radiology
University of Michigan
Ann Arbor, Michigan

**Ronald L. Eisenberg,
M.D.**
Clinical Professor of
    Radiology
University of California
    School of Medicine
San Francisco, California
University of California
    School of Medicine
Davis, California

Chairman of Radiology
Alameda County Medical
    Center
Oakland, California

Richard M. Gore, M.D.
Professor of Radiology
Northwestern University
    Medical School

Chief, Section of
    Gastrointestinal Radiology
Evanston Hospital-McGaw
    Medical Center of
    Northwestern University
Evanston, Illinois

Hedvig Hricak, M.D.,
Ph.D.
Professor of Radiology,
    Urology and Radiation
    Oncology

Chief, Abdominal Imaging
    Section
University of California
    School of Medicine
San Francisco, California

Martin J. Lipton, M.D.
Professor and Chairman
Department of Radiology
The University of Chicago
The University of Chicago
    Hospitals
Chicago, Illinois

Alexander R.
Margulis, M.D., DSc (hon)
Professor of Radiology
University of California
    School of Medicine
San Francisco, California

Charles E. Putman,
M.D.
James B. Duke Professor of
    Radiology
Professor of Medicine
Duke University Medical
    Center
Executive Vice President for
    Administration
Duke University
Durham, North Carolina

Donald Resnick, M.D.
Professor of Radiology
University of California, San
    Diego

Chief, Osteoradiology Section
Veterans Administration
    Medical Center
San Diego, California

Edward A. Sickles,
M.D.
Professor of Radiology
Chief, Breast Imaging Section
University of California
    School of Medicine
San Francisco, California

Preface

Medical imaging has made spectacular advances in the past fifteen years, reflecting the explosive developments in computers, electronics, and television. New cross-sectional imaging modalities are now widely used for diagnosing a broad spectrum of clinical disorders. Ultrasound is the most available and least expensive of these new techniques, but it is highly operator-dependent and requires rigorous training of technologists and physicians. Computed tomography is extremely versatile and has better signal-to-noise ratios than ultrasound. However, it is more expensive, uses ionizing radiation, and often requires the use of iodinated contrast media. Magnetic resonance imaging is the most sophisticated of these cross-sectional techniques, offering the best soft-tissue contrast resolution and the ability to image directly in multiple planes with a variety of pulse sequences. However, it is the most expensive and time-consuming of these imaging modalities. Nuclear medicine procedures now provide metabolic as well as morphological information, especially when using highly sophisticated tomographic procedures (SPECT, PET). The major disadvantage of nuclear medicine procedures is the need for the handling and disposal, the administration to patients, and in the case of PET, the very high cost of radioactive materials.

The availability of a wide variety of alternative imaging approaches comes at a time when the medical profession is facing severe financial constraints. Thus, it is essential that the practicing physician and resident-in-training have an understanding of the advantages and limitations of the newer (and the traditional) imaging procedures and a conception of their relative costs.

To meet this critical need, we have developed the *Radiology Pocket Reference* to recommend the most efficient and cost-effective imaging strategies for 300 clinical problems. The book is organized to reflect the two basic situations that the clinician faces when ordering an imaging study. The first part of each section deals with those symptoms and signs that do not permit a single working diagnosis. The second part provides coherent strategies that can be used when there is a working clinical diagnosis to be confirmed, refined, or rejected by imaging procedures. For every symptom or sign, a list of differential diagnoses is offered; for each clinical diagnosis, there is a brief outline of typical signs and symptoms as well as predisposing factors.

Our guiding principle in selecting the order of imaging examinations has been the need to combine cost effectiveness and noninvasiveness with high diagnostic accuracy. However, the reader must always take into consideration such local conditions as the availability and adequacy of equipment and the expertise of the radiologists performing the recommended studies. Therefore, we often suggest alternative approaches to be taken when modern equipment and adequate expertise are not available.

To fit the goal of a pocket-sized book that would receive frequent use, we have used a terse outline approach, choosing to include more clinical scenarios at the expense of long explanations. We intentionally did not burden the reader with detailed statistical information on sensitivity, specificity, accuracy, and positive and negative predictive values, because these figures vary greatly, are often in dispute, and are constantly changing. Similarly, we chose not to include specific references that would have made the book substantially longer without providing any additional practical information. Nevertheless, we have taken a wealth of experimental data into account in selecting those procedures that provide the highest likelihood of leading to the diagnosis.

To ensure that the information provided to the reader is up to date, each chapter has been edited by a prominent radiologist subspecializing in that area (in most instances the author of a highly regarded textbook in the field). Rather than repeat the same information throughout the book, we have included an appendix that describes the basics of each of the newer sophisticated imaging modalities as well as the relative costs of individual procedures in multiples of the basic chest radiograph.

We sincerely hope that the pocket-sized format of the book will make it readily available when it is needed most—in the many clinical situations in which there is not enough time to go to the medical library and consult larger, more encyclopedic texts. We intend to keep this reference book current by adding or deleting information as it becomes available in the literature. To meet our overall goal, we would appreciate receiving suggestions from readers concerning ways in which we could make this pocket-sized reference book even more user friendly.

Ronald L. Eisenberg, M.D.
Alexander R. Margulis, M.D.

Contents

CHEST

Charles E. Putman

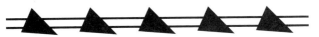

▶ SIGNS AND SYMPTOMS

Cough
Cyanosis
Dyspnea
Hemoptysis

Pleurisy
Stridor
Upper Airway Obstruction
Wheezing

▶ DISORDERS

Abscess (Lung)
Adult Respiratory
    Distress Syndrome
Asbestosis
Asthma
Atelectasis
Bronchiectasis
Bronchogenic Carcinoma
Bronchopleural Fistula
Chronic Bronchitis
Emphysema
Empyema
Hypersensitivity Lung
    Disease
Infectious Granulomatous
    Disease
Mediastinal Mass
  Anterior
  Middle

  Posterior
  Superior
Metastases (Pulmonary)
Pleural Effusion
Pneumoconioses
Pneumomediastinum
Pneumonia
Pneumonia in AIDS
Pneumothorax
Proper Tube Placement
Pulmonary Edema
Pulmonary Embolism
Pulmonary Fibrosis
Pulmonary Nodule
Sarcoidosis
Trauma (Blunt Chest)
Wegener's
    Granulomatosis

Cough

Common Causes

Inflammatory (laryngitis, tracheitis, bronchitis, bronchiolitis, pneumonia, lung abscess)

Mechanical (compression of airway due to neoplasm, foreign body, granulomas, bronchospasm)

Inhalation of particulate material (pneumoconioses)

Chemical (inhalation of irritant fumes, including cigarette smoke)

Thermal (inhalation of cold or very hot air)

Approach to Diagnostic Imaging

▶ I. **Plain chest radiograph**
   ▶ Preferred screening technique to demonstrate infection, neoplasm, or diffuse pulmonary parenchymal disease

Notes: Additional imaging studies are rarely needed except for appropriate follow-up radiographs (because the overwhelming majority of patients with clinically significant new cough will have pneumonia, bronchitis, or some other acute infectious disease of the respiratory tract).

Because a negative chest radiograph does not exclude a pneumonia (or cancer), especially in the immuno-compromised patient, if an antibiotic-sensitive infection is suspected clinically a sputum specimen should be obtained and the patient treated despite the unrevealing film.

Cyanosis

Presenting Signs and Symptoms

Bluish discoloration of the skin or mucous membranes (due to excess of reduced hemoglobin in the blood)

Common Causes

Impaired pulmonary function (pneumonia, pulmonary edema, chronic obstructive pulmonary disease)

Anatomic vascular shunting (congenital heart disease, pulmonary arteriovenous fistula)

Decreased oxygen in inspired air (high altitude)

Abnormal hemoglobin

Approach to Diagnostic Imaging

▶ I. **Plain chest radiograph**

   ▶ Preferred screening technique to demonstrate underlying pulmonary or cardiac abnormality

Dyspnea

Presenting Signs and Symptoms

Shortness of breath
Difficulty breathing on exertion
Uncomfortable awareness of breathing (increased muscular effort required)

Common Causes

Physical exertion
Hypoxia (high altitude)
Restrictive lung disease (pulmonary fibrosis, chest wall deformity)
Obstructive lung disease (emphysema, asthma)
Congestive heart failure
Pulmonary embolism

Approach to Diagnostic Imaging

▶ I. **Plain chest radiograph**
  ▶ Best screening technique for identifying an underlying pulmonary or cardiac cause (and any need for appropriate additional imaging studies)

Note: Soft-tissue views of the neck (or fiberoptic examination) may be helpful in patients with suspected acute upper airway obstruction.

Hemoptysis

Presenting Signs and Symptoms

Coughing up blood (resulting from bleeding from the respiratory tract)

Common Causes

Infection (pneumonia, tuberculosis, fungus, lung abscess)
Bronchogenic carcinoma
Bronchiectasis
Bronchitis
Pulmonary infarction (secondary to embolism)
Congestive heart failure

Approach to Diagnostic Imaging

▶ 1. **Plain chest radiograph**
   - ▸ Initial screening procedure
   - ▸ Normal study does not exclude neoplasm or bronchiectasis as the cause of the bleeding

▶ 2. **Fiberoptic bronchoscopy**
   - ▸ Indicated in the patient with a high clinical suspicion of malignancy and a relevant abnormality on the plain chest radiograph
   - ▸ Relatively invasive procedure with potential complications (e.g., hemorrhage, pneumothorax, hypoxemia)

▶ 3. **Computed tomography**
   - ▸ Indicated in the patient with a normal chest radiograph in whom the clinical suspicion of malignancy is relatively low
   - ▸ Indicated if a neoplasm is not detected by fiberoptic bronchoscopy (which is unreliable in locating peripheral tumors demonstrable by CT)

 Caveat: Despite a systematic and intensive search, the cause of hemoptysis will not be found in 30–40% of cases.

Pleurisy

Presenting Signs and Symptoms

Pain that is aggravated by breathing or coughing (may be of sudden onset, chronic, or recurring)

Rapid and shallow respiration

Limited motion of the affected side

Decreased breath sounds on the affected side

Pleural friction rub (characteristic finding that is often absent and frequently heard only 24–48 hours after the onset of pain)

Common Causes

Pneumonia

Tuberculosis

Pulmonary embolism

Trauma

Neoplasm

Occult rib fracture

Congestive heart failure

Mixed connective tissue disease

Pancreatitis

Approach to Diagnostic Imaging

▶ 1. **Plain chest radiograph**

  ▶ Preferred screening technique that may demonstrate the underlying pulmonary, rib, or chest wall abnormality as well as a confirming pleural effusion

Stridor

Presenting Signs and Symptoms

Musical sound that is predominantly inspiratory and is loud enough to be heard without a stethoscope at some distance from the patient (heard better over the neck than over the chest)

Common Causes

Upper airway obstruction
Epiglottitis
Croup
Inhaled foreign body
Pharyngeal tumor
Glottic edema
Retropharyngeal abscess

Approach to Diagnostic Imaging

▶ I. **Plain radiograph of the neck (soft-tissue technique)**
  ▶ Preferred screening technique to demonstrate narrowing or luminal obstruction of the upper airway (lateral projection is often more valuable than the frontal view)

Note: Laryngoscopy or CT of the neck may be required, especially in older patients in whom malignancy is more common and infection is a less likely cause.

Upper Airway Obstruction

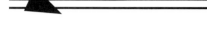

Presenting Signs and Symptoms

Musical sound that is predominantly inspiratory and is loud enough to be heard without a stethoscope at some distance from the patient (heard better over the neck than over the chest)

Common Causes

Epiglottitis
Croup
Inhaled foreign body
Pharyngeal tumor
Glottic edema
Retropharyngeal abscess

Approach to Diagnostic Imaging

▶ 1. **Plain radiograph of the neck (soft-tissue technique)**
  ▶ Preferred screening technique to demonstrate narrowing or luminal obstruction of the upper airway (lateral projection is more valuable than the frontal view)

Note: Laryngoscopy or CT of the neck may be required, especially in older patients in whom malignancy is more common and infection is a less likely cause.

Wheezing

Presenting Signs and Symptoms

Wheezing or whistling noise associated with breathing (implies obstruction to the flow of air at some level in the respiratory tract)

Most commonly heard on expiration

Common Causes

Asthma

Congestive heart failure

Pneumonia

Bronchogenic tumor

Pulmonary embolus

Foreign body

Approach to Diagnostic Imaging

▶ 1. **Plain chest radiograph**
   - ▶ Preferred screening study to exclude a tumor or a foreign body

Abscess (Lung)

Presenting Signs and Symptoms

Cough productive of moderate-to-large amounts of purulent, often foul-smelling sputum that may be tinged with blood

Fever and sweats

Chest pain and dyspnea

Anorexia and weight loss

Leukocytosis

Approach to Diagnostic Imaging

▶ 1. **Plain chest radiograph**
   - ▶ Preferred screening technique to demonstrate an area of consolidation that may develop into a cavity with an air-fluid level after rupture of the abscess into the bronchial tree
   - ▶ May permit differentiation of a peripheral lung abscess (round, formation of an acute angle with the chest wall) from an empyema (lenticular shape, formation of an obtuse angle with the chest wall)

▶ 2. **Computed tomography**
   - ▶ Best modality for differentiating peripheral lung abscess from empyema

---

Note: Most lung abscesses can be treated with antibiotic therapy and postural drainage; empyemas require a drainage procedure.

▶ 3. **Fiberoptic bronchoscopy**
   - ▶ May allow the removal of an underlying foreign body or excessive mucus and permit material to be obtained for culture

Adult Respiratory Distress Syndrome (ARDS)

Presenting Signs and Symptoms

Tachypnea, then dyspnea (24–48 hrs after initial illness/injury)
Noncardiogenic pulmonary edema
Hypoxemia and cyanosis

Common Causes

Diffuse pulmonary infection (bacterial or viral)
Aspiration of gastric contents
Direct chest trauma
Prolonged or profound shock
Inhalation of toxins and irritants
Systemic reaction to nonpulmonary processes (e.g., gram-negative septicemia, hemorrhagic pancreatitis, fat embolism)
Massive blood transfusion
Cardiopulmonary bypass ("pump lung")
Narcotic overdose pulmonary edema
Burns
Near-drowning

Approach to Diagnostic Imaging

▶ I. **Plain chest radiograph**
  ▶ Nonspecific diffuse bilateral opacities similar to pulmonary edema (but cardiac silhouette remains within normal size and there is no pleural effusion)
  ▶ Chest radiographic findings may lag many hours behind functional changes and appear much less severe than the clinical degree of hypoxemia
  ▶ Required during mechanical ventilation to detect evidence of barotrauma (pneumothorax, pneumomediastinum) and to evaluate tube placements (endotracheal, chest, and nasogastric tubes; Swan-Ganz catheter; central venous line)

Asbestosis

Presenting Signs and Symptoms

Insidious onset of exertional dyspnea and reduced exercise tolerance

Symptoms of airways disease (cough, sputum, wheezing) occurring primarily in heavy smokers

Common Causes

Occupational exposure

Approach to Diagnostic Imaging

▶ 1. **Plain chest radiograph**

    ▶ Preferred screening technique; may demonstrate irregular or linear small opacities (usually most prominent in the lower zones), characteristic diffuse or localized pleural thickening (pleural plaques), and calcification of the parietal pleura

    ▶ Relatively low specificity because of frequent difficulty in differentiating pleural thickening from normal intercostal muscles and extrapleural fat companion shadows of the chest wall (more likely asbestos-related if bilateral, symmetric, and along the midlateral chest wall)

▶ 2. **Computed tomography**

    ✓ ▶ High-resolution studies are superior to chest radiography for detecting pleural plaques

    ▶ Not recommended as a screening examination because of its high cost (good-quality chest radiographs interpreted by an informed reader have a high sensitivity and negative predictive value in the diagnosis of pleural plaques)

    ▶ Valuable for eliminating false-positive diagnoses of noncalcified plaques caused by muscle or fat, and for distinguishing pleural plaques from lung

Asthma

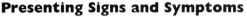

Presenting Signs and Symptoms

Episodic respiratory distress, often with tachypnea, tachycardia, and audible wheezes

Anxiety and struggling for air

Use of accessory muscles of respiration

Hyperexpansion of the lung (due to air trapping)

Prolonged expiratory phase

Approach to Diagnostic Imaging

► I. **Plain chest radiograph**
   ► Findings vary from entirely normal to hyperinflation, increased lung opacities, bronchial wall thickening, and regions of atelectasis

    Caveat: Once the diagnosis of asthma is established, chest radiographs are only required during recurrent episodes when there is clinical suspicion of complications (e.g., pneumothorax, atelectasis, secondary infection).

Atelectasis

Presenting Signs and Symptoms

Depend on the speed of the bronchial occlusion, the extent of lung affected, and the presence of infection

Note: Hypoxemia may cause decreased perfusion and produce a ventilation-perfusion mismatch.

Common Causes

Mucous plugs (tenacious bronchial exudate)
Endobronchial tumor
Granuloma
Foreign body
Extrinsic compression of a bronchus (enlarged lymph nodes, tumor, aneurysm)
External compression of the lung (pleural effusion, pneumothorax)
Neonatal respiratory distress syndrome (decreased or abnormal surfactant)
Infection (resorptive atelectasis)

Approach to Diagnostic Imaging

▶ 1. Plain chest radiograph
  ▶ Preferred screening technique to demonstrate characteristic linear streaks (plate-like atelectasis) or a segment of shrunken, airless lung
  ▶ If the atelectasis involves a substantial amount of the lung, the chest radiograph may show secondary elevation of the ipsilateral hemidiaphragm; shift of the trachea, heart, and mediastinum toward the affected area; and modification of the normal pulmonary vascular pattern
  ▶ May show the underlying cause of atelectasis (extrinsic mass, pleural effusion, pneumothorax)

▶ 2. **Fiberoptic bronchoscopy or computed tomography**
   ▶ Indicated to search for a cause of obstruction if there is no other obvious source for a collapsed segment or lobe

---

Note: Fiberoptic bronchoscopy may be therapeutic as well as diagnostic (e.g., removal of mucous plugs, obtaining material for culture or cytology).

Bronchiectasis

Presenting Signs and Symptoms

Chronic cough with sputum production (often after severe pneumonia with incomplete clearing of symptoms)

Hemoptysis

Recurrent pneumonia

Chronic atelectasis

Common Causes

Recurrent or chronic pneumonia

Chronic aspiration

Cystic fibrosis

Allergic bronchopulmonary aspergillosis

Interstitial pulmonary fibrosis

Tuberculous scarring (upper lobes)

Intrinsic bronchial disease (stenosis, extrinsic compression, endobronchial mass)

Approach to Diagnostic Imaging

▶ I. **Plain chest radiograph**
  ▶ Although more often normal, there may be increased interstitial opacities from recurrent inflammatory or infectious responses or changes consistent with subsegmental atelectasis
  ▶ Often "tram tracking" (parallel linear shadows representing the walls of cylindrically dilated bronchi) and areas of multiple thin-walled cysts, with or without air-fluid levels, which tend to be peripheral and cluster together in the distribution of a bronchovascular bundle

► **2. High-resolution computed tomography**
  ✓ ► High accuracy for demonstrating characteristic multiple, dilated, thin-walled circular lucencies (on cross section) and parallel linear opacities (bronchial walls sectioned lengthwise)
  ► Mucoid impactions may simulate lung nodules or branching, finger-like opacities
  ✓ ► Cystic bronchiectasis produces a "cluster of grapes" appearance

---

Note: CT has all but eliminated the need for contrast bronchography, except for those few patients considered for curative resection who appear to have localized disease according to CT.

► **3. Fiberoptic bronchoscopy**

Bronchogenic Carcinoma

Presenting Signs and Symptoms

Cough (with or without hemoptysis)
Dyspnea, wheezing, pneumonia
✓Weight loss
✓ History of smoking
Pleural effusion
Recurrent Horner's syndrome
Superior vena cava syndrome
Symptoms relating to distal metastases (e.g., occult fracture, seizure)

Note: May be an asymptomatic pulmonary nodule discovered incidentally on routine chest radiograph.

Risk Factors

Cigarette smoking
Occupational exposure (e.g., asbestos, radiation, arsenic, chromates, nickel, mustard gas)
Pulmonary scars (e.g., old inflammatory disease such as tuberculosis)

Approach to Diagnostic Imaging

▶ 1. **Chest radiograph**
  ▶ Preferred screening technique to show a solitary pulmonary nodule, atelectasis, pulmonary opacity, bronchial narrowing, hilar or mediastinal lymphadenopathy, pleural effusion

▶ 2. **Computed tomography**
  ▶ Permits percutaneous fine-needle biopsy of peripheral lesions to obtain material for cytologic studies

Staging

▶ 1. **Computed tomography (chest/upper abdomen)**

  ▶ Definitive noninvasive study to detect hilar and mediastinal lymphadenopathy and bronchial narrowing

  ▶ May show metastases in the liver and adrenal glands

Note: MRI may be valuable for detecting vascular invasion and mediastinal spread of tumor, as well as for clarifying whether adrenal enlargement is due to metastases or a benign cause.

Bronchopleural Fistula

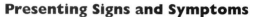

Presenting Signs and Symptoms

Fever, cough, dyspnea, and pleurisy
✓ Intractable pneumothorax
✓ Large air leak in a person with a pleural drain

Common Causes

Dehiscence of bronchial stump after lobectomy or pneumonectomy
Necrotizing pulmonary infection
Carcinoma of the lung with pleural invasion

Approach to Diagnostic Imaging

▶ 1. **Plain chest radiograph**
  ▶ Demonstrates a loculated intrapleural collection of air and fluid (with an air-fluid level on upright films)

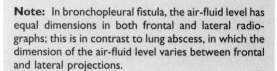

> **Note:** In bronchopleural fistula, the air-fluid level has equal dimensions in both frontal and lateral radiographs; this is in contrast to lung abscess, in which the dimension of the air-fluid level varies between frontal and lateral projections.

▶ 2. **Computed tomography**
  ▶ Can often distinguish a bronchopleural fistula from a peripheral lung abscess
  ▶ Occasionally may demonstrate the actual fistulous communication

▶ 3. **Sinogram**
  ▶ Injection of contrast material into a chest tube draining the pleural space may demonstrate the site of bronchial communication

Chronic Bronchitis

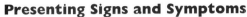

Presenting Signs and Symptoms

Chronic productive cough (excessive tracheobronchial mucus secretion sufficient to cause cough with expectoration of sputum that occurs on most days for at least 3 consecutive months in at least 2 consecutive years)

Common Causes

Cigarette smoking
Occupational exposure
Air pollution and other types of bronchial irritation
Chronic pneumonia
Superimposed emphysema

Approach to Diagnostic Imaging

▶ 1. **Plain chest radiograph**
  ▸ Normal examination in about half the patients
  ▸ May demonstrate nonspecific appearance with prominence of interstitial markings and thickened bronchial walls

---

Note: Chronic bronchitis is a clinical and not a radiographic diagnosis. Once the diagnosis of chronic bronchitis is established, chest radiographs are only required if there is clinical suspicion of a supervening acute pneumonia or a developing malignancy.

Emphysema

Presenting Signs and Symptoms

Exertional dyspnea (gradually progressive)
Productive cough
Abnormal pulmonary function tests

Common Causes

Cigarette smoking
Occupational exposure
α_1-antitrypsin deficiency
Congenital

Approach to Diagnostic Imaging

► I. **Plain chest radiograph**
  ► Although the lungs often appear normal in early stages of the disease, eventually there is hyperexpansion of the lungs (depressed diaphragm, generalized radiolucency of the lungs, enlarged retrosternal air space, ability to see diaphragmatic insertions on the ribs) and focal opacifications due to atelectasis or scarring
  ► Bullous changes (especially in the apices and subpleural regions)
  ► Marked attenuation and stretching (even virtual absence) of pulmonary vessels
  ► Often evidence of pulmonary hypertension (enlargement of central pulmonary arteries with rapid peripheral tapering)
  ► In α_1-antitrypsin deficiency, the emphysematous changes predominantly involve the lower lobes

 Caveat: Once the diagnosis of emphysema is established, repeat chest radiographs are only indicated if there is clinical indication of supervening disease (e.g., infection, congestive failure).

► 2. **Computed tomography**
  ► Although more sensitive than conventional radiography for detecting emphysematous changes in the lungs, this modality is rarely necessary. The extent of clinical derangement generally is determined by pulmonary function tests.
  ► CT is of special value in detecting otherwise unsuspected blebs and bullae in select high-risk populations, such as those with suspected α_1-antitrypsin deficiency or those who present with recurrent pneumothoraces

Empyema

Presenting Signs and Symptoms

Chest pain (varies from vague discomfort to stabbing pain and is often worse with coughing or breathing)
Rapid, shallow breathing
Fever, chills, and night sweats
Cough
Weight loss

> **Note:** If an empyema develops during the course of antibiotic treatment for bacterial pneumonia, the symptoms may be mild and the condition may go unrecognized.

Common Causes

Acute pneumonia
Lung abscess
Thoracic surgery or trauma
Spread from extrapulmonary sites (osteomyelitis of spine, subphrenic abscess)
Sepsis
Tuberculosis

Approach to Diagnostic Imaging

▶ I. **Plain chest radiograph**
  ▶ Preferred screening technique
  ▶ May permit differentiation of empyema (lenticular shape, formation of an obtuse angle with the chest wall) from lung abscess (round, formation of an acute angle with the chest wall)

►**2. Computed tomography**
  ► Best modality for differentiating empyema from peripheral lung abscess

> **Note:** Empyemas require a drainage procedure; most lung abscesses can be treated with antibiotic therapy and postural drainage.

  ► May show contrast enhancement of the parietal and visceral pleura, thickening of the extrapleural subcostal tissues, and increased attenuation of the extrapleural fat that are rarely seen with transudative effusions

►**3. Thoracentesis**
  ► Because a delay in diagnosis may have serious consequences, the patient with a suspected empyema requires thoracentesis for confirmation. Ultrasound can serve as a valuable guide for obtaining fluid from a loculated empyema.

Hypersensitivity Lung Disease

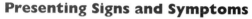

Presenting Signs and Symptoms

Range from mild respiratory symptoms and low fever (and prompt recovery) to severe pulmonary symptoms in a life-threatening condition

Striking blood eosinophilia (20–40% or more)

Coexistent bronchial asthma

Common Causes

Drug-induced eosinophilic lung disease (penicillin, aminosalicylic acid, hydralazine, chlorpropamide, sulfonamides)

Hypersensitivity pneumonitis (extrinsic allergic alveolitis)

Asthmatic pulmonary eosinophilia (hypersensitivity bronchopulmonary aspergillosis)

Tropical eosinophilia (parasites such as roundworms, filaria)

Pulmonary eosinophilia (Loffler's syndrome)

Approach to Diagnostic Imaging

▶ I. Plain chest radiograph
  ▶ Preferred screening technique for detecting the broad spectrum of pulmonary abnormalities seen in these disorders

Infectious Granulomatous Disease

Presenting Signs and Symptoms

Varies from asymptomatic exposure to fever, productive cough, and night sweats

Common Causes

Tuberculosis (especially in HIV–positive patients and in immigrants from Asia and Central America)

Histoplasmosis (central and eastern United States)

Coccidioidomycosis (southwestern United States and Mexico)

Blastomycosis (south-central and midwestern United States)

Cryptococcosis

Actinomycosis

Nocardiosis

Approach to Diagnostic Imaging

▶ I. **Plain chest radiograph**

　▶ Preferred screening technique to show the various patterns of opacifications within the lung (lobar consolidation; nodular opacities ranging from miliary to more discrete nodules; masses suggesting neoplasm; and diffuse disease with or without pleural effusion)

　▶ Best imaging modality for identifying potential complications (empyema, extensive atelectasis, and focal or diffuse dissemination of the primary disease)

Mediastinal Mass (Anterior)

Presenting Signs and Symptoms

Asymptomatic and incidental finding on plain chest radiograph

Myasthenia gravis (in up to 30–50% of patients with thymoma)

Common Causes

Thymoma

Teratoma

Lymphoma

Parathyroid tumor (ectopic)

Aortic aneurysm (ascending portion)

Morgagni hernia

Approach to Diagnostic Imaging

▶ 1. **Plain chest radiograph**
   - ▸ Detects and determines precise compartment of a mediastinal mass but otherwise does little to characterize the mass (can demonstrate erosion of the sternum in Hodgkin's disease and gas within a Morgagni hernia)

▶ 2. **Computed tomography**
   - ▸ Definitive imaging study for defining the origin and extent of the mass and for determining its underlying characteristics
   - ▸ With contrast enhancement, highly accurate in differentiating among fatty, cystic, and soft-tissue masses and aneurysms

▶ **3. Magnetic resonance imaging**
  - Equivalent to CT in confirming the presence and location of a mediastinal mass
  - Less effective than CT for assessing tracheal involvement and demonstrating calcification
  - Superior to CT for distinguishing tumor from fibrosis and in patients in whom the use of iodinated contrast material is contraindicated

Mediastinal Mass (Middle)

Presenting Signs and Symptoms

Asymptomatic and incidental finding on plain chest radiograph

Compression of trachea or esophagus (dysphagia, stridor, cough, wheezing, or localized or diffuse chest pain—depends more on size of mass than on its identity)

Common Causes

Lymph node enlargement (metastases, lymphoma, tuberculosis, histoplasmosis, sarcoidosis, pneumoconiosis

Aortic aneurysm

Dilated venous structures (azygos, hemiazygos, superior vena cava)

Bronchogenic carcinoma

Bronchogenic cyst

Pericardial cyst

Mediastinal hemorrhage/inflammation/lipomatosis

Approach to Diagnostic Imaging

▶ 1. **Plain chest radiograph**
   - ▶ Detects and determines precise compartment of a mediastinal mass but does little to characterize it

▶ 2. **Computed tomography**
   - ▶ Definitive imaging study for determining the origin and extent of the mass and for determining its underlying characteristics
   - ▶ With contrast enhancement, highly accurate in differentiating among fatty, cystic, and soft-tissue masses and aneurysms

► **3. Magnetic resonance imaging**
  ► Equivalent to CT in confirming the presence and location of a mediastinal mass
  ► Less effective than CT for assessing tracheal involvement by a mass and for demonstrating calcification
  ► Superior to CT for distinguishing tumor from fibrosis and in patients in whom the use of iodinated contrast material is contraindicated
  ► Ability to image directly in the coronal or sagittal plane is an advantage in those mediastinal regions that are parallel to the axial plane (subcarinal space, aortopulmonary window) and thus suffer from partial volume averaging effects on CT

 Caveat: **False-positive results may occur because of the relatively low spatial resolution of MRI, which may result in an inability to distinguish between a group of normal-sized nodes and a single enlarged node.**

Mediastinal Mass
(Posterior)

Presenting Sign and Symptom

Asymptomatic and incidental finding on plain chest radiograph

Common Causes

Neurogenic tumor
Vertebral lesion (trauma, infection, tumor)
Esophageal lesion (dilatation, neoplasm, diverticulum, duplication cyst)
Hiatal hernia
Lymphoma
Aortic aneurysm (descending portion)
Bochdalek hernia

Approach to Diagnostic Imaging

▶ 1. **Plain chest radiograph**
  ▶ Detects and determines precise compartment of a mediastinal mass but otherwise does little to characterize the mass (can show bone erosion in neurogenic tumor or air in a hiatal or Bochdalek hernia)

▶ 2. **Barium swallow**
  ▶ Indicated if there is clinical suspicion of an esophageal lesion

▶ 3. **Computed tomography**
  ▶ Definitive imaging study for defining the origin and extent of the mass and for determining its underlying characteristics
  ▶ With contrast enhancement, highly accurate in differentiating among fatty, cystic, and soft-tissue masses and aneurysms

► **4. Magnetic resonance imaging**
- ► Equivalent to CT in confirming the presence and location of a mediastinal mass
- ► Less effective than CT for showing calcification
- ► Superior to CT for showing the spinal cord and in patients in whom the use of iodinated contrast material is contraindicated

Mediastinal Mass (Superior)

Presenting Signs and Symptoms

Asymptomatic and incidental finding on plain chest radiograph

Displacement, deviation, or compression of the trachea (upper thoracic portion)

Common Causes

Substernal thyroid

Lymph node enlargement

Parathyroid mass

Other causes of anterior, middle, or posterior mediastinal masses

Approach to Diagnostic Imaging

▶ 1. **Plain chest radiograph**
  ▶ Detects a mass displacing, deviating, or compressing the trachea but otherwise does little to characterize the mass

▶ 2. **Radionuclide thyroid scan**
  ▶ Most accurate method for diagnosing the presence of abnormal thyroid tissue in the neck or superior mediastinum

▶ 3. **Computed tomography**
  ▶ Definitive imaging study for defining the origin and extent of the mass and for determining its underlying characteristics

▶ 4. **Magnetic resonance imaging**
- ▶ Equivalent to CT in confirming the presence and location of a mediastinal mass
- ▶ Less effective than CT for assessing tracheal involvement and for demonstrating calcification
- ▶ Superior to CT for distinguishing tumor from fibrosis and in patients in whom the use of iodinated contrast material is contraindicated

Metastases (Pulmonary)

Presenting Signs and Symptoms

Most are asymptomatic and only detected incidentally
during staging or follow-up of patients with known
malignancy

Develop in up to a third of patients with cancer

Only demonstrable metastases site in about half of patients with metastatic spread of tumor

Common Primary Sites of Tumor

Breast
Lung
Kidney
Thyroid
Head and neck
Melanoma

Approach to Diagnostic Imaging

▶ 1. **Plain chest radiograph**
  ▶ Preferred screening technique (detects almost all
    metastases greater than 15 mm in diameter)
  ▶ May fail to detect smaller nodules (because of over-
    lying ribs or blood vessels) and nodules in spe-
    cific areas (lung apices, inferior recesses just
    above dome of diaphragm, subpleural region)

▶ 2. **Computed tomography**
  ▶ Often detects small (3–10 mm), otherwise occult
    metastases (especially those located peripherally
    and in the subpleural region)
  ▶ Unfortunately, high sensitivity of CT leads to po-
    tential problem of false-positive examinations
    (granulomas, intrapulmonary lymph nodes, or
    even pulmonary vessels on end are sometimes
    erroneously interpreted as metastases)
  ▶ Best imaging modality for following the response of
    metastases to chemotherapy

> **Note:** Although resolution of nodules indicates a positive response, persistent nodular opacities representing sterilized tumor deposits may be seen after successful treatment of metastatic seminoma, choriocarcinoma, or hypernephroma.

▶ 3. **Radionuclide thyroid scan (total body)**
> ▶ Highly specific and more sensitive than plain chest radiographs for detecting thyroid carcinoma metastatic to the lung

Indications for CT if Plain Chest Radiograph Is Normal

▶ 1. High propensity of tumor spread to lung (melanoma, testicular carcinoma, choriocarcinoma, head and neck tumors)

▼ **Caveat:** Common primary tumors of the lung, breast, colon, prostate, and cervix have a low propensity of spread to the lungs.

▶ 2. Presence of metastases would alter treatment (usually by cancellation of planned extensive surgery).
> ▶ Radical amputation for osteosarcoma
> ▶ Extensive lymph node dissection for melanoma
> ▶ Lobectomy for presumed solitary metastasis or several nodules localized to one lobe

▶ 3. Effective therapy available for metastases (osteogenic sarcoma, choriocarcinoma, nonseminomatous testicular tumors, renal cell carcinoma, certain functioning thyroid carcinomas)

▼ **Caveat:** The detection of pulmonary metastases is of no clinical significance if there is no effective treatment for metastases or if there already are obvious extrathoracic metastases.

Pleural Effusion

Presenting Signs and Symptoms

Pleuritic pain

Dyspnea

Often asymptomatic and discovered as incidental finding
on chest radiograph

Decreased or absent breath sounds, percussion dullness,
and decreased motion of hemithorax

Common Causes

Congestive heart failure (usually bilateral but larger on
right)

Neoplasm (primary or metastatic lung cancer, lymphoma)

Pneumonia

Ascites

Pancreatitis (usually left-sided)

Tuberculosis

Pulmonary embolism (small)

Mixed connective tissue disease (lupus, rheumatoid arthritis)

Trauma (hemothorax)

Approach to Diagnostic Imaging

▶ **1.** **Plain chest radiograph**
  - ▶ Preferred screening technique that can show classic blunting or meniscus appearance at the lateral and posterior costophrenic angles, apical cap, or increased opacity of the hemithorax without obscuration of vascular markings
  - ▶ Large effusions may opacify an entire hemithorax and cause shift of the mediastinum to the opposite side
  - ▶ Subpulmonic effusions may be detected by an unusually lateral position of the top of the diaphragmatic contour on supine films
  - ▶ Lateral decubitus projection (affected side down) can determine whether pleural fluid is free or loculated and estimate the amount of the effusion

▶ **2.** **Computed tomography**
  - ▶ Procedure of choice for determining the status of the underlying lung parenchyma in a patient with extensive pleural effusion (e.g., may detect lung abscess, pneumonia, or bronchogenic carcinoma that is hidden from view on plain radiograph)
  - ▶ Limited value in differentiating transudates from exudates or chylous effusions

▶ **3.** **Ultrasound**
  - ▶ Readily available for bedside imaging in severely ill patients in whom a lateral decubitus projection cannot be obtained
  - ▶ Best technique for identifying and localizing a loculated effusion as an echo-free or hypoechoic fluid collection separate from the lung and chest wall that may mimic a mass on plain radiographs
  - ▶ May permit demonstration of an exudate as a complex, septated pattern or a homogeneously echogenic appearance
  - ▶ Permits marking of the chest wall for thoracentesis (may be performed under ultrasound guidance in difficult cases)

Pneumocomioses

Presenting Signs and Symptoms

Insidious onset of decreased pulmonary function (related to occupational exposure to inorganic dusts)

Common Types

Silicosis
Asbestosis
Coal worker's pneumoconiosis
Talcosis

Approach to Diagnostic Imaging

▶ 1. **Plain chest radiograph**
  ▶ Preferred screening technique that may demonstrate a broad spectrum of chronic changes in the lung parenchyma and pleura

> **Note:** There may be poor correlation between the extent of radiographic findings and the degree of alteration in pulmonary function.

▶ 2. **Computed tomography**
  ▶ Although CT is more sensitive than plain chest radiography for detecting subtle changes, this modality is not usually necessary for clinical evaluation

Pneumomediastinum

Presenting Signs and Symptoms

Chest pain
May be asymptomatic

Common Causes

Spontaneous
Trauma (injury to chest wall, bronchus, trachea, or lung)
Iatrogenic (surgery or instrumentation of the esophagus, trachea, bronchi, or neck; overinflation during anesthesia and respiratory therapy)
Extension of gas from the neck or abdomen
Asthma (primarily in children)
Rupture of the esophagus (e.g., Boerhaave's syndrome)
Hyaline membrane disease (extension of pulmonary interstitial emphysema)

Approach to Diagnostic Imaging

▶ I. **Plain chest radiograph**
  ▸ Preferred imaging technique for detecting gas separating the medial margin of the pleura from the mediastinal contents or interposed between the heart and diaphragm
  ▸ Can show any associated pneumoperitoneum or gas within the soft tissues of the neck

---

Note: The clinical concern in patients with pneumomediastinum is the possible development of a pneumothorax, which can have dire consequences in patients whose respiratory status is already compromised.

Pneumonia

Presenting Signs and Symptoms

Cough with sputum production
Fever and chills
Chest pain and dyspnea

Predisposing Factors

Viral respiratory infection
Cigarette smoking
Chronic obstructive pulmonary disease
Alcoholism
Unconsciousness
Dysphagia with regurgitation
Hospitalization or institutionalization
Surgery/trauma
Heart failure
Immunosuppressive disorders and therapy

Approach to Diagnostic Imaging

▶ I. **Plain chest radiograph**
  ▶ Preferred screening technique to show the various patterns of opacifications within the lung
  ▶ Best imaging modality for identifying potential complications (empyema, extensive atelectasis, and focal or diffuse dissemination of the primary infection)

Notes: The mere presence of an opacity in a patient with fever or chest pain does not necessarily indicate the presence of an infectious process. Atelectasis, neoplasm, pulmonary embolism or infarction, and atypical pulmonary edema can all mimic pneumonia both clinically and radiographically.

Pneumonia may exist in the presence of a normal radiograph (especially with atypical organisms and those pneumonias that develop in the immunocompromised host).

Frequent radiographs after acute pneumonia in the *normal* population should *not* be obtained (unnecessary cost and radiation exposure) unless there is some clinical reason to warrant serial studies. Symptoms usually resolve even though the radiographic opacity may be unchanged and persistent. However, in the *immunocompromised* patient in whom clinical manifestations may be depressed, serial chest radiographs are justified as they may be the only means of following the results of a course of therapy.

▶ **2. Computed tomography**
  ▶ May be indicated if there is incomplete clearing of an opacity or if there is clinical suspicion of either postobstructive pneumonia distal to an endobronchial lesion or a secondary lung abscess

Pneumonia in AIDS Patients

Presenting Signs and Symptoms

Cough with sputum production
Fever and chills
Chest pain and dyspnea

Predominant Organisms

Pneumocystis carinii
Histoplasmosis
Cytomegalovirus
Cryptococcosis
Aspergillosis
Toxoplasmosis
Varicella

Approach to Diagnostic Imaging

▶ I. **Plain chest radiograph**
   - ▶ Preferred screening technique to show the various patterns of opacifications within the lung
   - ▶ Best imaging modality for identifying potential complications (empyema, extensive atelectasis, and focal or diffuse dissemination of the primary infection)

Notes: The mere presence of an opacity in a patient with fever or chest pain does not necessarily indicate the presence of an infectious process. Atelectasis, neoplasm, pulmonary embolism or infarction, and atypical pulmonary edema can all mimic pneumonia both clinically and radiographically.

The radiograph may be normal even though there is clinical evidence of pneumonia. Conversely, in immuno-compromised patients, there may be extensive radiographic findings with minimal clinical manifestations. Therefore, in this population serial chest radiographs are justified in that they may be the only means of following a course of therapy (as opposed to the normal population, in which frequent radiographs after acute pneumonia should not be obtained).

Pneumothorax

Presenting Signs and Symptoms

Range from asymptomatic to sudden sharp chest pain, severe dyspnea, shock, and life-threatening respiratory failure

Pain may be referred to corresponding shoulder, across the chest, or over the abdomen (simulating acute coronary occlusion or acute abdomen)

Markedly depressed or absent bowel sounds

Shift of mediastinum to opposite side (with large or tension pneumothorax)

Common Causes

Spontaneous (rupture of small, usually apical bleb)

Trauma (penetrating, blunt, rib fracture)

Complication of mechanical ventilation (barotrauma)

Chronic obstructive pulmonary disease

Chronic pulmonary disease (e.g., sarcoidosis, eosinophilic granuloma)

Pneumocystis carinii pneumonia

Lung abscess with bronchopleural fistula

Rupture of the esophagus

Extension from pneumomediastinum

Iatrogenic (surgery, lung or pleural biopsy, thoracentesis, central line placement)

Approach to Diagnostic Imaging

▶ I. Plain chest radiograph

    ▶ Preferred screening technique that shows apical and lateral air without peripheral lung markings and separated from normal lung by a sharp pleural margin

    ▶ May show underlying bullous or interstitial changes consistent with chronic obstructive pulmonary disease or any chronic interstitial lung disorder

Notes: Pneumothorax is best seen on an *expiration* film obtained with low penetration (light film).

In patients on mechanical ventilation for adult respiratory distress syndrome, a small pneumothorax on a supine film may present subtly as a loculated collection in a subpulmonic or paracardiac location and be associated with a pneumomediastinum.

Caveat: The visceral pleural line of a pneumothorax may be mimicked by skin folds (resulting from compression of redundant skin by the radiographic cassette). The key is to identify normal vascular markings that extend peripherally beyond the skin fold interface. The visceral pleural line may also be mimicked by bullae (it is necessary to detect the thin curvilinear walls that are concave rather than convex to the chest wall).

▶ **2. Computed tomography**
- ▶ Although CT is more sensitive than plain chest radiographs for detecting a pneumothorax, this modality is rarely necessary
- ▶ May be required to differentiate pneumothorax from bullous disease and in patients in whom an anterior pneumothorax is suspected on a supine radiograph but who cannot undergo upright or lateral decubitus films

Proper Tube Placement

Indication for Study

Determination of the tip of a radiopaque tube placed within the thorax

Common Types of Tubes

Endotracheal tube
Central venous pressure (CVP) catheter
Swan-Ganz catheter
Nasogastric tube

Approach to Diagnostic Imaging

▶ 1. **Plain chest radiograph**
  ▶ Demonstrates whether the tip of the tube is in the proper position
  ▶ **Endotracheal tube:** With the head in a neutral position, tip should be 5–7 cm above the carina

---

Note: With flexion and extension of the neck, the tip of the tube will move about 2 cm caudally and cranially, respectively.

  ▶ **Central venous pressure catheter:** Within the superior vena cava (above the level of the right atrium)

Note: Up to a third of CVP catheters are incorrectly placed at the time of initial insertion.

▸ **Swan-Ganz catheter:** Within the right or left main pulmonary arteries

---

Note: Too peripheral a position of the tip may lead to occlusion of the pulmonary artery and resulting distal pulmonary infarction.

▸ **Nasogastric tube:** Stomach

Note: The tip of the tube may remain in the esophagus above the esophagogastric junction or be misplaced in the bronchial tree.

Pulmonary Edema: Cardiac vs. Noncardiac (Permeability)

Types of Edema

▶ 1. **Cardiac**
  - ▶ Low-protein transudate due to increased hydrostatic pressure generated across the capillary membrane that initially accumulates in the connective tissues surrounding the blood vessels

▶ 2. **Noncardiac**
  - ▶ Protein-rich exudate that accumulates in the extravascular space as a consequence of increased microvascular permeability. Because of the high protein osmotic pressure of the extravasated proteins, water may not flow from the extravasation toward the loose connective tissue but may flood the alveolar space.

Note: Clearance of the protein-rich exudate is slower than that of the nonproteinaceous transudate.

Approach to Diagnostic Imaging

► I Plain chest radiograph

  ► Can distinguish between cardiac and noncardiac (permeability) edema in about 80% of cases using the following criteria:

	Cardiac	Noncardiac
Major Signs		
Kerley's lines	Present	Unusual
Pleural effusions	Present	Unusual
Cardiomegaly	Present	Unusual
Opacities in lung	Diffuse	Patchy and peripheral
Minor Signs		
Air bronchograms	Rare	Often present
Hilar haze	Present	Infrequent
Peribronchial cuffs	Present	Unusual

Pulmonary Embolism

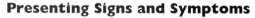

Presenting Signs and Symptoms

Nonspecific tachypnea, dyspnea, and hemoptysis

Major Risk Factors

Prolonged bed rest

Recent surgical procedure

Recent myocardial infarction or chronic congestive heart failure

Deep venous thrombosis in the veins of the pelvis or proximal lower extremities

Indwelling venous catheter

Approach to Diagnostic Imaging

▶ I. **Plain chest radiograph**

- ▶ Usually normal (may be nonspecific opacity, pleural effusion, atelectasis, or elevation of the hemidiaphragm consistent with other pulmonary or pleural processes)

- ▶ Classic pleural-based, wedge-shaped opacity (Hampton's hump) is seen in a minority of cases with pulmonary infarction

- ▶ Uncommon findings of focal oligemia (Westermark's sign) and enlargement of the ipsilateral pulmonary artery (Fleischner's sign)

- ▶ Essential for accurate interpretation of radionuclide lung scan

▶ 2. Radionuclide ventilation-perfusion (V/Q) lung scan

 ▶ Preferred screening test for detecting clinically significant pulmonary emboli

 ▶ If the perfusion study is *normal*, significant embolization is excluded and no further studies are needed

 ▶ If segmental or larger perfusion defects are present with normal ventilation in these areas (V/Q mismatch), there is a high likelihood of pulmonary embolism

 Caveat: There may be a relatively large number of indeterminate examinations in patients with chronic pulmonary disease or parenchymal abnormalities on plain chest radiographs.

▶ 3. Pulmonary arteriography

 ▶ Most definitive study (gold standard) that shows pulmonary emboli as intraarterial filling defects or abrupt cut-off (complete obstruction) of pulmonary vessels

 ▶ Although it is an invasive procedure, pulmonary arteriography is indicated if the radionuclide scan is indeterminate or of intermediate probability and there is a clinical need for a definitive diagnosis

 ▶ Indicated to confirm a high probability radionuclide scan *only* if the patient is either a surgical candidate (for venous occlusion or embolectomy) or at extremely high risk for anticoagulation

Pulmonary Fibrosis

Presenting Signs and Symptoms

Often asymptomatic except for insidious onset of exertional dyspnea

Cough (if secondary bronchial infection)

Anorexia, weight loss, fatigue, weakness, and vague chest pains

Cyanosis, cor pulmonale, clubbing (severe disease)

Common Causes

Idiopathic (Hamman-Rich syndrome, UIP)

Collagen vascular diseases (scleroderma, rheumatoid arthritis)

Sarcoidosis

Eosinophilic granuloma

Occupational exposure

Immunosuppressive and antineoplastic drugs (busulfan, bleomycin, methotrexate, cyclophosphamide)

Approach to Diagnostic Imaging

▶ I. **Plain chest radiograph**

▶ Preferred screening technique to show characteristic pattern of prominent linear markings, rounded opacities, and small cystic lesions (honeycombing) as well as evidence of pulmonary hypertension and cor pulmonale

 Caveat: **Chest films may be normal even in the presence of significant symptoms or functional abnormalities.**

▶ 2. **Computed tomography**
  ▶ Although high-resolution CT is more sensitive than plain chest radiographs for detecting pulmonary fibrosis and suggesting the correct histologic diagnosis, this modality is not usually required in clinical practice

---

Note: Lung biopsy may be needed if the imaging findings and clinical course do not indicate the precise diagnosis.

Pulmonary Nodule (Solitary)

Presenting Signs and Symptoms

Asymptomatic
Incidental finding on a chest radiograph

Common Causes

Benign nonneoplastic process (granuloma, arterio-venous malformation)
Benign neoplastic process (hamartoma, bronchial adenoma)
Primary bronchogenic carcinoma
Solitary metastasis

Age Effect on Malignancy in Benign-Appearing Nodule (small, round, sharply defined)

Younger than age 30: Cancer risk is less than 1%
Ages 30 to 45: Cancer risk is about 15%
Older than age 50: Cancer risk is 50%

Radiographic Criteria for Benignancy

Central dense or popcorn calcification
No growth demonstrated on serial chest films over 2 years

Approach to Diagnostic Imaging

▶ 1. **Chest fluoroscopy (low kVp technique)**
  ▶ May detect characteristic benign calcification and thus obviate any further investigation
  ▶ May show that apparent nodule actually represents only a healing rib fracture or pleural changes

▶ 2. **Computed tomography**
- ▶ May show additional nodules not visible on plain chest radiograph (suggesting metastases)
- ▶ Detection of any hilar or mediastinal metastases
- ▶ Permits percutaneous fine-needle aspiration biopsy of peripheral lesions as an alternative to thoracotomy for establishing a definite diagnosis (25% pneumothorax rate, although chest tube required in only 5%; false-negative rate of about 10% in patients with carcinoma)

Sarcoidosis

Presenting Signs and Symptoms

Asymptomatic (hilar and mediastinal lymphadenopathy discovered incidentally on a routine chest radiograph)

Constitutional symptoms (fever, weight loss, anorexia, fatigue)

Erythema nodosum and other skin lesions

Uveitis

Hypercalcemia/hypercalciuria

Variety of symptoms involving the cardiac, respiratory, musculoskeletal, and central nervous systems

Common Causes

Unknown

Approach to Diagnostic Imaging

▶ 1. **Plain chest radiograph**
  ▶ Preferred screening technique that may demonstrate characteristic bilateral hilar and right paratracheal lymphadenopathy and a diffuse reticular pulmonary infiltration that may accompany or follow the lymphadenopathy

▶ 2. **Computed tomography**
  ▶ High-resolution studies are more sensitive than plain chest radiographs for detecting the parenchymal pulmonary changes as well as enlarged lymph nodes in regions that are invisible on plain radiographs

Note: Although good correlation has been shown between the CT findings and pulmonary function, clinically this imaging modality is not as important as the response to therapy and pulmonary function tests.

Trauma (Blunt Chest)

Approach to Diagnostic Imaging

▶ 1. **Plain chest radiograph**
   ▶ Preferred initial screening study that can confirm suspected clinical diagnoses (tension pneumothorax, hemothorax, pulmonary contusion) and can diagnose or suggest other injuries that may be difficult to detect by clinical examination (mediastinal and pericardial hemorrhage; diaphragmatic rupture; and bronchial, esophageal, or pulmonary parenchymal laceration)
   ▶ May be obtained during acute resuscitation efforts

▶ 2. **Computed tomography**
   ▶ Far more sensitive than plain chest radiography for detecting pneumothorax, ruptured diaphragm or esophagus, pleural or pericardial hemorrhage, and pulmonary contusion and laceration
   ▶ Although controversial, CT may be effective in demonstrating mediastinal hemorrhage and determining the need for aortography to exclude aortic rupture in a patient with a limited indication for aortography (based on the reported mechanism of injury) or whose plain chest radiographs are equivocal or of suboptimal quality

Note: An unequivocally normal CT scan of the mediastinum may indicate that the aorta is intact and thus preclude the need for aortography.

▶ 3. **Aortography**
   ▶ Immediately required in patients with history of blunt decelerating thoracic injury and radiologic evidence of mediastinal hemorrhage

Wegener's Granulomatosis

Presenting Signs and Symptoms

Paranasal sinus congestion and pain

Nasal mucosal ulcerations (with consequent secondary
bacterial infection)

Serous or purulent otitis media with hearing loss

Cough, hemoptysis, dyspnea, and pleuritis

Glomerulonephritis (renal failure is major cause of
death)

Common Causes

Unknown

Approach to Diagnostic Imaging

▶ 1. **Plain chest radiograph**
- ▶ Preferred screening technique to demonstrate the
  characteristic multiple and bilateral thick-walled
  cavitating lung lesions (50% of patients) as well
  as a pattern of diffuse or nodular opacities that
  may simulate metastases

▶ 2. **Computed tomography**
- ▶ Best imaging technique for detecting mucosal and
  submucosal lesions in the tracheobronchial tree
  (seen almost exclusively in women) that produce irregular narrowing of the airway lumen

CARDIOVASCULAR
Martin J. Lipton

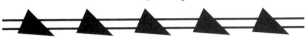

▶ SIGNS AND SYMPTOMS

Angina Pectoris
Claudication

Congestive Heart Failure
Peripheral Ischemia
   (Acute)

▶ DISORDERS

Heart
Cardiac Tumors
Cardiomyopathy
  Congestive
  Hypertrophic
  Restrictive

Congenital Heart Disease
Cor Pulmonale
Endocarditis (Infective)
Myocardial Infarction
Valvular Heart Disease

Pericardium
Cardiac Tamponade
Constrictive Pericarditis

Pericardial Effusion

Vascular
Aneurysm
  Abdominal Aorta
  Peripheral
  Thoracic Aorta
Aortic Dissection
Deep Venous Thrombosis

Peripheral Occlusive
   Vascular Disease
Superior Vena Cava
   Syndrome
Thoracic Outlet
   Syndrome

Angina Pectoris

Presenting Signs and Symptoms

Episodes of precordial discomfort or pressure, typically precipitated by exertion and relieved by rest or sublingual nitroglycerine

Common Cause

Atherosclerotic coronary artery disease

Risk Factors

Elevated serum cholesterol
High cholesterol intake
Tobacco smoking (cigarettes primarily)
Diabetes mellitus
Hypertension
Strong family history

Approach to Diagnostic Imaging

► I. Radionuclide myocardial perfusion scan
  ► SPECT scanning has a specificity and sensitivity approaching 95% for detecting areas of myocardial ischemia as perfusion defects on stress testing that fill in during an examination performed with the patient at rest

---

Note: Perfusion defects that are stable during both stress and rest examinations usually represent areas of infarction.

▶ **2. Coronary arteriography**
  ▸ Indicated when angioplasty or bypass surgery is being considered to evaluate the extent and severity of disease (percentage of stenosis involving one, two, or three vessels)
  ▸ Left ventricular angiogram can be performed to evaluate wall motion (if not contraindicated by potential adverse effects of additional volume of contrast material on renal or ventricular function

> **Note:** Wall motion can also be assessed by radionuclide techniques or echocardiography.

▶ **3. Radionuclide gated blood pool studies**
  ▸ To evaluate the ejection fraction because of the important relationship between ventricular function and prognosis

▶ **4. Angioplasty**
  ▸ Interventive technique in which inflation of a balloon-tipped catheter at the site of a stenotic atherosclerotic lesion can rupture the intima and media and dramatically dilate the obstruction

> **Note:** This is an alternative to bypass grafting in the patient with suitable anatomic lesions (risk is comparable to surgery).

Evaluating Postsurgical Patency of Bypass Grafts

▶ **1. Ultrafast computed tomography or magnetic resonance imaging**
  ▸ Accuracy of more than 90% for establishing patency of coronary artery bypass grafts

Claudication

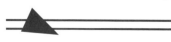

Presenting Signs and Symptoms

Deficient blood supply to muscles during exercise (initially intermittent, may proceed to continuous pain at rest)

Common Cause

Atherosclerotic vascular disease

Approach to Diagnostic Imaging

▶ **1. Ultrasound with color Doppler**
  ▶ Preferred noninvasive screening technique to demonstrate the presence of atherosclerotic plaques and assess the degree of stenosis of the lumen

▶ **2. Arteriography**
  ▶ Indicated if surgery or angioplasty is contemplated to define the location and extent of the lesion more precisely and to assess the status of the peripheral runoff vessels

> **Note:** Magnetic resonance angiography is rapidly improving and may eventually replace contrast arteriography for evaluating the peripheral vascular system.

▶ **3. Interventive radiology**
  ▶ Percutaneous transluminal angioplasty is an excellent alternative to surgery for dilating localized stenotic lesions (especially in the iliac arteries where the success rate approaches 95%)

> **Note:** The success rate in arteries of the thigh and calf is about 50–60%.

Congestive Heart Failure

Common Causes

Left ventricular failure
Valvular heart disease (stenosis or regurgitation)
Pulmonary venoocclusive disease
Congenital heart disease

Approach to Diagnostic Imaging

► **1. Plain chest radiograph**

- ► Demonstrates classic findings of indistinct vascular markings, progressive redistribution of venous blood flow to the lungs (cephalization), and Kerley B lines (edematous thickening of the interlobular septa at the periphery of the lungs)

► **2. Echocardiography**

- ► Indicated to evaluate the dimensions of the left ventricle and other cardiac chambers, ejection fraction, wall motion dysfunction, and the presence and severity of incompetence or stenosis of the heart valves
- ► Echo and color Doppler studies can accurately detect the presence of pericardial effusion, intracardiac thrombi, and cardiac tumors

Peripheral Ischemia (Acute)

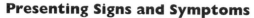

Presenting Signs and Symptoms

Sudden onset of severe pain, coldness, numbness and pallor of a portion of an extremity

Absent pulses distal to the obstruction

Common Causes

Embolization (from the heart, a proximal atherosclerotic plaque, or an aneurysm)

Acute thrombosis on preexisting atherosclerotic disease

Approach to Diagnostic Imaging

▶ I. **Arteriography**

 ▶ Demonstrates the precise site of obstruction and permits therapeutic thrombolysis of the clot

  Caveat: Lytic therapy is contraindicated in patients with active bleeding; recent gastrointestinal bleeding, central nervous system surgery, or stroke; intracranial tumor; or nonviable extremity. Complications include bleeding, puncture site hematoma, pericatheter thrombus formation, and distal embolization.

Cardiac Tumors

Presenting Signs and Symptoms

Protean findings of fever, elevated erythrocyte sedimentation rate, anemia, weight loss, syncope, and embolic symptoms

Left atrial lesions may mimic rheumatic valvular disease

Common Causes

Myxoma

Rhabdomyoma, lipoma, fibroma

Sarcoma

Metastases (breast, lung, lymphoma, melanoma)

Approach to Diagnostic Imaging

▶ 1. **Echocardiography (especially transesophageal)**
   - ▶ In left atrial myxoma, confirms the presence of a filling defect that often prolapses into the left ventricle during diastole

▶ 2. **Magnetic resonance imaging**
   - ▶ In the patient with a suspected malignant cardiac tumor, MRI is excellent for detecting direct extension of the lesion, intracardiac metastases, and pericardial involvement

▶ 3. **Computed tomography**
   - ▶ Indicated for demonstrating invasion of the heart by noncardiac tumors of the lung or mediastinum
   - ▶ Electron-beam CT is diagnostic of most intracardiac masses (including blood clots)

Cardiomyopathy (Congestive)

Presenting Signs and Symptoms

Congestive heart failure (may be right-sided or left-sided dominance or biventricular involvement)

Common Causes

Chronic diffuse myocardial ischemia (coronary artery disease)

Infection (especially Coxsackie virus, Chagas disease)

Toxins or drugs (ethanol, Adriamycin*, cocaine, psychotherapeutic drugs)

Granulomatous disease (sarcoidosis, giant cell myocarditis, Wegener's granulomatosis)

Metabolic disease (endocrinopathies, lipid or glycogen storage diseases, uremia)

Nutritional deficiencies (beriberi, selenium deficiency, kwashiorkor)

Connective tissue disorders

Approach to Diagnostic Imaging

▶ I. **Plain chest radiograph**
   ▸ Demonstrates global cardiomegaly and evidence of congestive failure

---

Note: Detection of coronary artery calcification may be a clue to an underlying ischemic cause.

---

*Adria Laboratories, Columbus, OH

▶ 2. **Echocardiography, radionuclide scan, magnetic resonance imaging, or electron-beam computed tomography**
  ▶ Echocardiography shows dilated, hypokinetic cardiac chambers with reduced fractional shortening while excluding primary valvular disease or segmental wall motion abnormalities (seen in discrete myocardial infarcts)
  ▶ Gated myocardial scintigraphy demonstrates abnormal ejection fractions and times; gallium scanning can detect acute myocarditis
  ▶ MRI shows dilatation of specific cardiac chambers, abnormal ejection fractions and stroke volumes, and an abnormal texture of the myocardial tissue. If available, MRI is excellent for assessing all types of cardiomyopathy (including asymmetric septal hypertrophy that can be difficult to define completely using echocardiography).

Cardiomyopathy (Hypertrophic)

Presenting Signs and Symptoms

Chest pain
Syncope
Palpitations
Exer ional dyspnea
Congestive heart failure

> **Note:** Sudden death occurs in about half the patients (overall mortality rate about 2–3% per year).

Common Causes

Familial (autosomal dominance with variable penetration)
Obstructive (subaortic or midventricular)

Approach to Diagnostic Imaging

▶ 1. **Plain chest radiograph**
  ▶ Deceptively normal-looking in about 50% of cases (because hypertrophy occurs at the expense of the ventricular cavities)
  ▶ May demonstrate left atrial enlargement (commonly due to mitral regurgitation)
  ▶ May show right ventricular enlargement or an unusual shape of the cardiac silhouette that is not diagnostic of any specific disorder (e.g., neither a valvular lesion nor pericardial effusion)

▶ 2. **Echocardiography**
  ▶ Preferred noninvasive modality that permits measurement of the thickened ventricular walls and allows differentiation among the different subgroups
  ▶ Often permits quantitation of the degree of obstruction of the outflow tract (an important determinant of the effectiveness of treatment)

▶ 3. **Electron-beam computed tomography**
  ▶ If available, permits diagnosis and quantitation of the severity of hypertrophic cardiomyopathy (allows assessment of all areas of the myocardium and is not subject to the imaging limitations of echocardiography)
  ▶ May evaluate left ventricular mass and provide indices of left ventricular function, as well as exclude other cardiac and noncardiac abnormalities

Cardiomyopathy (Restrictive)

Presenting Signs and Symptoms

Congestive heart failure
Arrhythmias
Heart block

Common Causes

Infiltrative disorders (amyloid, glycogen storage disease, mucopolysaccharidoses, hemochromatosis, sarcoidosis, tumor infiltration of the myocardium)
Endomyocardial fibrosis (highly prevalent in tropics)

Approach to Diagnostic Imaging

▶ 1. **Plain chest radiograph**
  ▸ Typically shows a normal-sized (or even small) heart with pulmonary venous congestion

▶ 2. **Echocardiography or magnetic resonance imaging**
  ▸ Shows normal systolic and diastolic function, myocardial hypertrophy, and often dilatation of the atria
  ▸ Demonstrates a normal pericardium, thus permitting differentiation from constrictive pericarditis (in which the pericardium is thickened)
  ▸ T2-weighed MR images show high signal in the myocardium in patients with amyloidosis or sarcoidosis

► **3. Electron-beam computed tomography**

> ► Highly accurate in differentiating restrictive cardio-myopathy from constrictive pericarditis

 Caveat: Limited use in patients with severe congestive heart failure, in whom contrast material is best avoided.

Congenital Heart Disease

Presenting Signs and Symptoms

Broad spectrum of murmurs, shunts, alterations in systemic and pulmonary blood flow, and altered work loads of specific cardiac chambers

Cyanosis (in right-to-left shunts)

Risk Factors

Chromosomal defects (trisomy 13, 18, 21; Turner's syndrome; Holt-Oram syndrome)

Maternal illness (diabetes mellitus, systemic lupus erythematosus)

Environmental exposure (e.g., thalidomide)

History of congenital heart disease in a first-degree relative

Common Types

Atrial septal defect

Ventricular septal defect

Patent ductus arteriosus

Total anomalous venous return

Persistent truncus arteriosus

Transposition

Endocardial cushion defect

Tetralogy of Fallot

Hypoplastic right heart syndrome

Coarctation of the aorta

Approach to Diagnostic Imaging

BEFORE BIRTH

▶ **1. Prenatal ultrasound**
  ▶ May permit the diagnosis of some serious defects during pregnancy (thus offering the parents the option of discontinuing the pregnancy or permitting the physician and parents to make realistic plans for the labor, delivery, and care of the child)

AFTER BIRTH

▶ **1. Plain chest radiograph**
  ▶ Initial screening study for assessing the pulmonary vascularity, size of the main pulmonary artery, size and position of the aorta (especially whether it is right-sided), and size and contour of the cardiac silhouette

▶ **2. Echocardiography**
  ▶ Plays a prominent role in the initial imaging evaluation of congenital heart disease

▶ **3. Magnetic resonance imaging**
  ▶ Cine studies have become the primary modality for imaging most congenital heart disease because of the ability to show directly both morphologic and functional anomalies in multiple planes

> **Note:** Electron-beam CT can provide similar information, but it currently is less available.

▶ **4. Angiocardiography**
  ▶ Definitive (but invasive) study

> **Note:** Some authors recommend angiocardiography only if surgery is contemplated.

Cor Pulmonale

Presenting Signs and Symptoms

Exertional dyspnea
Angina pectoris
Syncope

Common Causes

Chronic obstructive pulmonary disease
Pulmonary fibrosis
Acute or chronic pulmonary embolism
Primary pulmonary hypertension
Pulmonary venoocclusive disease
Extrapulmonary diseases affecting pulmonary mechanics (morbid obesity, chest wall deformities, neuromuscular disease)

Approach to Diagnostic Imaging

▶ 1. **Plain chest radiograph**
  ▶ Although radiography usually shows a normal-sized heart or only mild cardiomegaly, there may be enlargement of the right ventricle and right atrium

---

Note: Plain films may be relatively insensitive indicators of right ventricular enlargement because hyperinflation of the lungs and bullae may distort the position of the heart in these patients.

▸ Characteristic prominence of the main and central pulmonary arteries with rapid tapering (pruning) such that the lung periphery appears oligemic

---

Note: The lungs usually will show evidence of chronic obstructive pulmonary disease or interstitial fibrosis (i.e., right ventricular failure is secondary to pulmonary arterial or parenchymal disease).

▸**2. Echocardiography or radionuclide studies**

▸ Indicated to evaluate the degree of function of the left ventricle (as well as the degree of enlargement of the right atrium and right ventricle)

Endocarditis (Infective)

Presenting Signs and Symptoms

Insidious onset of low-grade fever, night sweats, fatigue, malaise, weight loss

New regurgitant murmur and signs of valvular insufficiency

Chills and arthralgia

Emboli may produce stroke, myocardial infarction, flank pain and hematuria, abdominal pain, or acute arterial insufficiency in an extremity.

Petechial hemorrhages and Osler's nodes

Predisposing Factors

Rheumatic heart disease

Congenital heart disease (ventricular septal defect, tetralogy of Fallot)

Prosthetic heart valve

Intravenous drug abuse

Central venous line

Approach to Diagnostic Imaging

▶ I. **Echocardiography**
  ▶ Procedure of choice for demonstrating the characteristic vegetations on affected heart valves

---

Notes: Transesophageal studies can increase the specificity and sensitivity of echocardiography from about 60% to 90% and are indicated if the diagnosis remains in question after conventional echocardiography.

Echocardiography should be repeated after 6 weeks of intravenous antibiotic therapy for infective endocarditis.

►**2. Electron-beam computed tomography**
- ► Demonstrates not only the vegetations but also valvular calcification, distorted orifices, and aneurysms of the sinus of Valsalva
- ► A complementary procedure to echocardiography, especially in seriously ill patients who cannot lie flat (i.e., the table can be tilted)

Note: Infections of prosthetic valves can result in perivalvular or perisutural leaks that may be detected by cine MRI.

Myocardial Infarction

Presenting Signs and Symptoms

Deep substernal chest pain (described as an aching or pressure) that often radiates to the back, jaw, or left arm

Pain is similar to that of angina pectoris but is usually more severe, long lasting, and relieved only a little or briefly by rest or nitroglycerine

Symptoms of left ventricular failure, pulmonary edema, shock, or significant arrhythmia may dominate the clinical appearance

About 20% of acute myocardial infarctions are silent (or not recognized as an illness by the patient)

Elevation of myocardial enzymes in the serum

 Caveat: In some cases, acute chest pain may suggest possible aortic dissection (see page 94).

Common Cause

Atherosclerotic coronary artery disease

Approach to Diagnostic Imaging

▶ I. **Plain chest radiograph**
   ▶ Simple, inexpensive screening technique that is useful as a baseline for assessing pulmonary venous congestion

Direct Infarct Imaging

 Caveat: The diagnosis of myocardial infarction is usually evident from the patient's history and confirmed by electrocardiogram and enzyme studies. Infarct imaging is indicated if the clinical, laboratory, and electrocardiographic findings are equivocal; if there has been recent cardiac surgery or trauma; or if there is a suspicion of right ventricular infarction.

▶ 1. **Radionuclide imaging, electron-beam computed tomography, or magnetic resonance imaging**
   ▶ Can demonstrate areas of myocardial infarction and usually can determine whether they are acute or remote

---

Note: Echocardiography is often performed to assess the function of the right and left ventricles as well as to detect the 10–20% incidence of cardiac-wall clots that alter the clinical management.

Valvular Heart Disease

Presenting Signs and Symptoms

Murmur and clinical symptoms vary depending on the precise valve involved and whether there is predominant stenosis or regurgitation

Common Causes

Rheumatic fever
Congenital heart disease
Infectious endocarditis

Approach to Diagnostic Imaging

▶ 1. **Plain chest radiograph**
  ▶ Inexpensive screening technique to show enlargement of the entire heart or specific chambers, valvular calcification, and any evidence of pulmonary vascular congestion

▶ 2. **Echocardiography**
  ▶ More precisely demonstrates any chamber enlargement or wall thickening and the precise size of the orifices of affected valves
  ▶ Doppler flow studies can assess the degree of regurgitation

---

Note: Although not yet widely used, cine MRI shows promise for demonstrating and quantitating the regurgitation of blood across any incompetent valve (without the need for contrast material).

Cardiac Tamponade

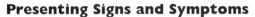

Presenting Signs and Symptoms

Cardiogenic shock (low cardiac output and low systemic arterial pressure)

Tachycardia

Dyspnea and orthopnea

Usually elevation of both systemic venous pressure (prominent neck veins) and pulmonary venous pressure

Distant heart sounds

Pericardial rub

Pulsus paradoxus (accentuation of the normal inspiratory decline in systemic systolic blood pressure greater than 10 mm Hg)

Mechanism

Pericardial effusion under tension causing compression of the cardiac chambers and compromising diastolic filling

Approach to Diagnostic Imaging

▶ 1. **Plain chest radiograph**
   ▶ Demonstrates rapid enlargement of the cardiac silhouette with relatively normal-appearing vascularity

▶ 2. **Echocardiography**
   ▶ Modality of choice not only to demonstrate the accumulation of a large amount of pericardial fluid but also to show septal shift, paradoxic septal motion, diastolic collapse of the right ventricle, and cyclical collapse of the atria

Constrictive Pericarditis

Presenting Signs and Symptoms

Elevation of ventricular diastolic, atrial, pulmonary, and systemic venous pressures (unlike tamponade the ventricular venous pressure, or ejection fraction, is usually preserved)

Dyspnea and orthopnea (prolonged elevation of pulmonary venous pressure)

Hypervolemia, engorgement of neck veins, pleural effusion, hepatomegaly, ascites, peripheral edema (elevated systemic venous pressure)

Kussmaul's sign (inspiratory swelling of neck veins), which is absent in tamponade

Common Causes

Postpericardiotomy (although the pericardium is usually partly resected after coronary artery bypass grafting)

Viral infection (especially Coxsackie-B)

Tuberculosis

Uremia

Radiation

Neoplastic involvement

Rheumatoid arthritis

Idiopathic

Approach to Diagnostic Imaging

▶ I. **Plain chest radiograph**
  ▶ Demonstrates characteristic pericardial calcification in 50% of cases (as well as pleural effusions, small atria, a flat or straightened right heart border, and dilated superior and inferior vena cava and azygos vein)

▶ 2. **Magnetic resonance imaging or computed tomography**
  ▶ Preferred screening techniques to show the abnormally thick pericardium (which permits the distinction of constrictive pericarditis from restrictive cardiomyopathy)

Notes: MRI is more specific in that it can show that the pericardial thickening represents fibrosis.

Although echocardiography can show the thickened pericardial wall, the findings are not as specific as in the case of pericardial fluid.

Pericardial Effusion

Presenting Signs and Symptoms

Severity of symptoms varies greatly depending on the underlying cause as well as the rate at which the pericardial fluid accumulates and the total amount present

Milder symptoms include chest pain and a friction rub; large effusions may lead to congestive heart failure and shock

Faint, distant heart sounds on auscultation

Common Causes

Idiopathic

Infection

Autoimmune (systemic lupus erythematosus, rheumatoid arthritis, scleroderma)

Dressler's and postpericardiotomy syndromes

Neoplasm (lymphoma, lung or breast metastases)

Drug-induced (procainamide, hydralazine, phenytoin)

Uremia

Myxedema

Congestive heart failure

Trauma

Approach to Diagnostic Imaging

► I. **Plain chest radiograph**

   ► Suggests the diagnosis if there is a rapid increase in the size of the cardiac silhouette on serial chest films (especially when the lungs remain clear)

Note: A rapid increase in heart size related to congestive heart failure is generally associated with pulmonary venous congestion.

▶ **2. Echocardiography**
   ▶ Procedure of choice for demonstrating as little as 50 mL of pericardial fluid (normal, 20 mL) as a posterior sonolucent collection

---

Note: CT is valuable for detecting loculated pericardial effusions, whereas MRI may be able to characterize the fluid as serous or hemorrhagic (because of characteristic changes in signal intensity).

Aneurysm
(Abdominal Aorta)

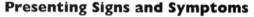

Presenting Signs and Symptoms

Most are asymptomatic and discovered incidentally on
routine physical examination or plain abdominal radiograph

Pulsatile mass

Severe abdominal pain and hypotension (if rupture)

Common Causes

Atherosclerosis

Trauma

Arteritis syndromes

Connective tissue disorders (Marfan's syndrome, cystic
medial necrosis)

Syphilis

Approach to Diagnostic Imaging

▶ I. **Ultrasound**

  ▸ Most cost-effective screening technique to show di-
    latation of the aorta to greater than 3 cm and the
    presence of intraluminal clot

  ▸ Serial examinations can be easily performed to fol-
    low aneurysm size in patients who are not con-
    sidered surgical candidates at the time

   Caveat: Limited ability of ultrasound to
  show consistently the proximal and distal extent of the aneurysm and its relationship to
  the surrounding retroperitoneal structures
  (required prior to elective surgical repair)

▶ **2. Computed tomography**
  ▸ Indicated if there is suspicion of retroperitoneal hematoma secondary to leaking or acute rupture
  ▸ Although CT is more accurate than ultrasound for determining the true diameter of an aneurysm and its longitudinal extent, it is more expensive and requires contrast material

---

Note: Helical CT with 3-dimensional reformatting permits demonstration of the abdominal aorta in multiple planes, improves the visualization of the relationship of an aneurysm to the origins of the renal arteries, and ensures a constant bolus of contrast material throughout the aorta.

▶ **3. Magnetic resonance imaging**
  ▸ Indicated only if ultrasound and CT fail to provide information about renal, visceral, and iliac artery involvement of an aneurysm
  ▸ MR angiography may eventually supplant catheter angiography in the preoperative assessment of abdominal aortic aneurysms

► **4. Aortography**

- ► Traditionally, the preoperative procedure of choice for determining the number of renal arteries and their relationship to the aneurysm, and the patency of the visceral, renal, external iliac, and femoral arteries (factors that may modify the surgical approach and define additional procedures required to decrease postoperative morbidity)

- ► Because aortography outlines only the aortic lumen, it underestimates the true size of an aneurysm if its wall is lined with thrombus.

Note: The ability of newer, less invasive techniques such as CT and MR angiography to demonstrate the extent of the aneurysm and the patency of other vessels has substantially reduced the need for preoperative aortography, which now is rarely required for this purpose.

 Caveat: There is *no* indication for plain lateral radiographs of the abdomen to detect calcification in the wall of an aneurysm (very low sensitivity).

Aneurysm (Peripheral)

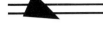

Presenting Signs and Symptoms

Limb ischemia (due to thrombus within the aneurysm)
Signs of distal embolization
Gangrene

Common Causes

Atherosclerosis
Trauma
Mycotic
Complication of vascular surgery

Approach to Diagnostic Imaging

▶ I. **Ultrasound with color Doppler**
  ▶ Preferred screening procedure for detecting a peripheral aneurysm (most commonly involving the popliteal artery) and assessing its size

---

Note: CT or MRI is generally required to assess subclavian artery aneurysms.

▶ 2. **Arteriography**
  ▶ Usually required prior to surgery (bypass grafting and aneurysm repair) to evaluate the status of the peripheral vessels

Aneurysm
(Thoracic Aorta)

Presenting Signs and Symptoms

Asymptomatic
Symptoms may be due to secondary compression
    Stridor, wheezing (trachea and bronchi)
    Dysphagia (esophagus)
    Venous obstruction of the upper extremities, head,
      and neck (superior vena cava)
    Hoarseness (recurrent laryngeal nerve)
May be substernal or back pain

Common Causes

Atherosclerosis
Syphilis
Mycotic
Connective tissue disorders (Marfan's and Ehlers-Danlos
    syndromes)

Approach to Diagnostic Imaging

▶ I. **Plain chest radiograph**
    ▶ Inexpensive screening study to demonstrate con-
      tour abnormalities and tortuosity of the thoracic
      aorta as well as calcification within its wall

 Caveat: It may be difficult to distinguish
a thoracic aneurysm from other mediastinal
masses.

► **2. Computed tomography or magnetic resonance imaging**
  ► These preferred methods for initial evaluation and follow-up of thoracic aneurysms can accurately demonstrate vessel diameter, mural thrombus, calcifications, degree of luminal patency, mass effects on adjacent mediastinal structures, and evidence of leakage or rupture
  ► CT is superior to MRI for showing calcifications within the wall of an aneurysm
  ► MRI is superior to CT for demonstrating the relationship of an aneurysm to the arch vessels (because of its ability to directly image in the sagittal plane) and requires no contrast material

---

Note: Transesophageal ultrasound is increasingly being used for accurately sizing thoracic aortic aneurysms, especially in unstable patients, since it can be rapidly performed at the bedside.

► **3. Aortography**
  ► Indicated only for preoperative planning when it is vital to know the relationship between the aneurysm and the great vessels and coronary arteries, as well as the vascular supply to the spinal cord

---

Note: Aortography is unreliable for assessing the size of an aneurysm as it only visualizes the patent portion of the lumen and cannot show the extent of mural thrombus.

Aortic Dissection

Presenting Signs and Symptoms

Sudden, severe, tearing substernal chest pain with radiation to the back

Frequent migration of pain from the original site as the dissection extends along the aorta

Aortic insufficiency murmur

Absent or asymmetric major arterial pulses

Neurologic complications (stroke, paraparesis, or paraplegia from spinal cord ischemia; ischemic peripheral neuropathy from abrupt occlusion of an artery supplying a limb)

Predisposing Factors

Hypertension

Connective tissue disorders (Marfan's and Ehlers-Danlos syndromes)

Bicuspid aortic valve

Coarctation of the aorta

Trauma

Granulomatous arteritis

Pregnancy (cause of half the dissections in women younger than age 40)

Previous aortic surgery or arterial catheterization

Approach to Diagnostic Imaging

▶ I. **Plain chest radiograph**
  ▶ Demonstrates mediastinal widening in up to 90% of patients and frequently a left pleural effusion
  ▶ Localized bulging of the aortic contour indicates the likely site of origin of a dissection

▶2. Computed tomography

- ▸ Preferred screening study in the acutely ill patient to show the classic double-barrel aorta (opacification of both the true and false lumen) and intimal flap (linear filling defect within the aortic lumen)

Note: If available, transesophageal ultrasound is also an extremely sensitive screening technique for diagnosing aortic dissection.

▶3. Magnetic resonance imaging

- ▸ Although probably the best noninvasive technique for imaging the aorta, MRI is often difficult to obtain in severely ill patients who require life-support systems and close monitoring

---

Note: Procedure of choice for the detection of chronic aortic dissections.

▶4. Aortography

- ▸ This most definitive study is required if surgical therapy is contemplated to identify precisely the origin and extent of the dissection, the severity of any aortic insufficiency, and the extent of involvement of major arterial trunks arising from the aorta (including the coronary arteries)

Deep Venous Thrombosis

Presenting Signs and Symptoms

Asymptomatic (one-third of patients with symptomatic pulmonary emboli but no clinical signs of DVT will nevertheless have a lower extremity venous thrombus)

Variable combination of pain, edema, warmth, skin discoloration, and prominent superficial veins over the involved area

Delayed complications of dermatitis, ulceration, and varicosities

Common Causes

Stasis (postoperative, postpartum states; chronic illness)

Pregnancy or the use of oral contraception

Obesity

Hypercoagulability (malignant tumor, blood dyscrasia)

Endothelial injury (indwelling catheter, injection of irritating substance, septic phlebitis, thromboangiitis obliterans)

Prolonged immobilization with the legs dependent while traveling (especially on prolonged airplane flights)

Approach to Diagnostic Imaging

► I. **Color Doppler ultrasound**
  ► Preferred screening modality (>95% accuracy) that can demonstrate lack of compressibility of the vein (indicating the presence of thrombus within it), visualization of the intraluminal thrombus itself, and characteristic alterations in spontaneous flow that occur because of obstruction of the proximal veins

►**2. Venography**
  ► Traditional gold standard that can demonstrate the conclusive finding of a persistent filling defect within the lumen of the vein
  ► Other findings that are highly suggestive of deep venous thrombosis include abrupt termination of the contrast column within the vein, inability to opacify a major vein, and the formation of extensive collateral venous circulation

---

Note: See the section on pulmonary embolus (page 52).

Peripheral Occlusive Vascular Disease

Presenting Signs and Symptoms

Intermittent claudication that progresses to pain at rest
Coolness and numbness of the affected extremity
Nonhealing ulcers
Gangrene
Diminished pulses distal to the area of narrowing

Vessels Primarily Involved

Superficial femoral artery
Aortoiliac system
Trifurcation vessels
Popliteal artery

Approach to Diagnostic Imaging

▶ 1. **Ultrasound with color Doppler**
  ▸ Preferred noninvasive screening technique to demonstrate the presence of atherosclerotic plaques and assess the degree of stenosis of the lumen

▶ 2. **Arteriography**
  ▸ Indicated if surgery or angioplasty is contemplated to define more precisely the location and extent of the lesion and to assess the status of the peripheral runoff vessels

Note: MR angiography is rapidly improving and may eventually replace contrast arteriography for evaluating the peripheral vascular system.

▶ **3. Interventive radiology**
  ▶ Percutaneous transluminal angioplasty is an excellent alternative to surgery for dilating localized stenotic lesions (especially in the iliac arteries where the success rate approaches 95%)

Note: The success rate in arteries of the thigh and calf is about 50–60%.

Superior Vena Cava Syndrome

Presenting Signs and Symptoms

Progressive dilatation of the veins of the head and upper
extremities
Edema and plethora of the face, neck, and upper torso
Cyanosis and conjunctival edema
Dizziness, syncope, and headache
Respiratory distress (due to airway edema)

Note: If the obstruction occurs slowly, the formation
of a compensatory collateral venous network may prevent the development of clinical symptoms.

Common Causes

Malignant neoplasm (primary bronchogenic carcinoma,
lymphoma, metastases from breast carcinoma)
Mediastinal granulomatous or fibrosing disease
Long-term indwelling central venous catheters
Aortic aneurysm

Approach to Diagnostic Imaging

▶ 1. **Computed tomography or magnetic resonance
imaging**
   ▶ Preferred noninvasive methods for showing both
the proximal dilatation of the superior vena cava
and its branches and the underlying cause of the
obstruction

▶ **2. Venography**
  ▶ Indicated only if there is a valid clinical need for more anatomic detail or functional hemodynamic assessment or as a preoperative procedure

---

Note: Percutaneous placement of a vascular stent is often used for treatment (especially in patients with end-stage renal failure).

Thoracic Outlet Syndrome

Presenting Signs and Symptoms

Numbness, paresthesias, pain, and sensory and motor deficits in the hand, neck, shoulder, or arm (secondary to arterial, venous, or nerve compression)

Obliteration of the radial pulse on the involved side with 90° elevation and external rotation of the arm or with simultaneous hyperextension of the neck and turning the head toward the affected side (if the artery is involved)

Intermittent cyanosis, edema, and thrombotic symptoms (if the vein is involved)

Common Causes

Congenital anatomic anomaly (cervical rib, abnormal insertion of the anterior scalene muscle on the first rib)

Aberrant healing of rib or clavicle fracture

Neoplasm

Approach to Diagnostic Imaging

▶ 1. **Plain chest radiograph**
   - ▶ Screening study for demonstrating a cervical rib or a tumor in the apex of the lung

▶ 2. **Arteriography or venography**
   - ▶ Studies performed in both the neutral position (arms at the sides) and in the position that reproduces the patient's symptoms may demonstrate kinking or partial obstruction of the subclavian artery or vein

GASTROINTESTINAL

Richard M. Gore

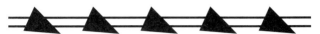

▶ SIGNS AND SYMPTOMS

Ascites
Constipation
Diarrhea
Dysphagia
Gastrointestinal Bleeding

Chronic, Origin
   Obscure
Acute Lower
Acute Upper
Jaundice
Nausea and Vomiting

▶ DISORDERS

Abscess

Peritonitis
Suspected Abdominal (No
   Localized Findings)
Hepatic
Left Subphrenic Space

Pancreas/Lesser Sac
Perihepatic
Pelvic
Renal/Perirenal
Splenic

Mass

Abdominal Mass in a
   Neonate
Abdominal Mass in a
   Child
Diffusely Enlarged
   Abdomen (No
   Discrete Mass)

Epigastric
Hypogastric
Left Lower Quadrant
Left Upper Quadrant
Midabdominal
Right Lower Quadrant
Right Upper Quadrant

Esophagus

Achalasia
Cancer
Diffuse Esophageal Spasm
Laceration (Mallory-Weiss
    Syndrome)
Perforation
Reflux Esophagitis
Scleroderma
Varices (Esophageal/
    Gastric)

Stomach/Duodenum

Cancer
Peptic Ulcer Disease
Zollinger-Ellison
    Syndrome

Small Bowel

Gastroenteritis
Obstruction

Colon

Antibiotic-Associated
    Colitis
Appendicitis
Cancer
Crohn's Disease
Ulcerative Colitis
Diverticulitis
Diverticulosis
Hemorrhoids
Irritable Bowel Syndrome
Obstruction

Liver/Biliary Tract

Cholecystitis
    Acute
    Chronic
Fatty Liver
Hemangioma
Hepatocellular Carcinoma
    (Hepatoma)
Metastases
Portal Hypertension

Pancreas

Pancreatitis
    Acute
    Chronic
Cancer

Trauma (Blunt Abdominal)

Ascites

Presenting Signs and Symptoms

Small amounts may be asymptomatic
Abdominal distension and discomfort
Anorexia, nausea, and early satiety
Respiratory distress (due to reduced lung volume)
Bulging flanks, fluid wave, shifting dullness

Common Causes

Cirrhosis
Neoplasm (hepatic cancer or peritoneal carcinomatosis)
Congestive heart failure
Tuberculosis (and other infections)
Hypoalbuminemia (nephrotic syndrome, protein-losing
enteropathy, malnutrition)

Approach to Diagnostic Imaging

▶1. **Ultrasound**
- ▶ Mobile, echo-free fluid regions shaped by adjacent
structures
- ▶ Smallest amounts (as little as 100 mL) in a supine
patient appear first around the inferior tip of the
right lobe of the liver, the superior right flank,
the cul-de-sac of the pelvis, and the hepatorenal
area (Morison's pouch)

▶2. **Computed tomography**
- ▶ Although more expensive, CT may demonstrate the
underlying abdominal disease process (if ultrasound fails to do so)
- ▶ May be able to distinguish ascites (water attenuation) from blood (higher attenuation) or chyle
(lower attenuation)

 Caveat: Plain abdominal radiographs are
not indicated because a large amount of
fluid (800–1000 mL) must be present to be
detected and the underlying cause is infrequently shown.

Constipation

Presenting Signs and Symptoms
Decrease in frequency of stools or difficulty in defecation

Common Causes

ACUTE
Bowel obstruction or adynamic ileus

CHRONIC
Neurologic dysfunction (diabetes, spinal cord disorder, Parkinsonism, idiopathic megacolon)

Scleroderma

Drugs (anticholinergic agents, opiates, aluminum-based antacids)

Hypothyroidism

Cushing's syndrome

Hypercalcemia

Debilitating infection

Anorectal pain (fissures, hemorrhoids, abscess, proctitis)

Approach to Diagnostic Imaging

▶ **1. Plain abdominal radiograph**
  ▸ Detects mechanical bowel obstruction

▶ **2. Barium enema**
  ▸ For better characterization of the site and cause of narrowing or obstruction of the bowel

▶ **3. Radiopaque marker study**
  ▸ A plain abdominal radiograph 5 days after ingesting the tablets can indicate whether there is a significant delay in clearing the radiopaque material from the bowel

▶ **4. Defecography (evacuation proctography)**
  ▸ Dynamic study that can demonstrate mechanical abnormalities such as rectal intussusception, anterior wall prolapse, and rectocele

Diarrhea

Presenting Signs and Symptoms

Increased volume, fluidity, or frequency of fecal discharges

Common Causes

Osmotic (lactase deficiency, polyvalent laxative abuse)

Secretory (viral or protozoal infection, bacterial toxins, castor oil, Zollinger-Ellison syndrome, prostaglandin therapy, vasoactive intestinal peptide

Exudative (mucosal inflammation, necrosis, neoplasm)

Malabsorption (sprue, pancreatic insufficiency, bowel resection, Whipple's disease)

Altered intestinal motility (diabetes, hyperthyroidism, magnesium-containing laxatives, irritable bowel syndrome)

Approach to Diagnostic Imaging

▶ I. **Small bowel study**

> ▶ May suggest underlying causes such as sprue or scleroderma (dilated small bowel), hypoproteinemia (regularly thickened folds), Whipple's disease (irregularly thickened folds), inflammatory bowel disease (ileitis or colitis), tuberculosis (ileocecal inflammation), intestinal fistula, motility disorders

 Caveat: Plain abdominal radiographs are *not* indicated.

Dysphagia

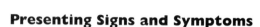

Presenting Signs and Symptoms

Difficulty initiating swallowing
Food sticking in the upper or middle esophageal region
Odynophagia (pain on swallowing)
Regurgitation
Aspiration

Common Causes

Carcinoma
Peptic or lye stricture
Achalasia
Scleroderma
Diffuse esophageal spasm
Cervical esophageal web
Lower esophageal (Schatski's) ring
Neuromuscular disorder

Approach to Diagnostic Imaging

▶ I. **Barium swallow** (imaged on video or fast-sequence radiographs)

   Caveat: Hyperosmolar water-soluble contrast should *not* be used because aspiration of this material causes increased fluid to enter the tracheobronchial tree and may lead to the development of pulmonary edema.

Gastrointestinal Bleeding (Chronic, Obscure Origin)

Presenting Signs and Symptoms

Anemia (iron deficiency)
Hematest/Guaiac positive stools

Common Causes

Neoplasm (benign or malignant anywhere in alimentary tube)
Peptic ulcer
Gastritis
Meckel's diverticulum
Angiodysplasia

Approach to Diagnostic Imaging

▶ 1. **Barium enema (double contrast)**
  ▶ If results are *negative* proceed to
▶ 2. **Upper gastrointestinal series (biphasic)**
  ▶ If results are *negative* proceed to
▶ 3. **Enterolysis (*not* a "small bowel follow through")**
  ▶ If results are *negative* proceed to
▶ 4. **Arteriography (celiac, SMA, IMA)**
  ▶ May detect a vascular malformation (angiodysplasia) or an occult neoplasm that is the underlying source of the bleeding
  ▶ If results are *negative* (especially in young patients) consider
▶ 5. **Radionuclide scan for Meckel's diverticulum**
  ▶ Isotope may collect in ectopic gastric mucosa

Note: Endoscopy and colonoscopy can also be used to detect a source of chronic gastrointestinal bleeding depending on the availability of physicians skilled in performing these techniques.

Gastrointestinal Bleeding
(Acute Lower)

Presenting Sign and Symptom

Brisk rectal bleeding without blood in gastric aspirate

Common Causes

Diverticulosis
Angiodysplasia
Ischemic colitis
Hemorrhoids (diagnosed by proctoscopy)
Polyps/carcinoma (more frequently associated with chronic bleeding)

Approach to Diagnostic Imaging

▶ I. **Radionuclide scan**

- ▶ Most sensitive diagnostic study that can document active bleeding as little as 0.05–0.1 mL/min as a focal area of increased radionuclide activity corresponding to extravasation of blood in the gastrointestinal tract

- ▶ Movement of the radionuclide proximally or distally indicates active bleeding. Lack of movement suggests an angiodysplasia, arteriovenous malformation, or vascular tumor.

Note: If the radionuclide scan shows no evidence of an active bleeding site, there is *no* indication for arteriography.

▶ **2. Arteriography**
  ▶ If bleeding continues to be rapid (>0.5–1 mL/min), arteriography may show the precise bleeding site by demonstrating extravasation of contrast material into the lumen of the bowel or the tangled blood vessels of an angiodysplasia
  ▶ Offers therapeutic options through transcatheter measures (embolization or vasoconstrictive agents) and may preclude the need for surgery (especially in diverticular hemorrhage)

Note: Many patients have a positive radionuclide scan and a bleeding site demonstrated surgically but a *negative* arteriogram.

▶ **3. Barium enema or colonoscopy**
  ▶ Indicated only if bleeding is minimal or has stopped, to search for underlying colonic pathology that *may* represent the bleeding site

Notes: Introduction of barium into the colon prevents the performance of arteriography until the barium has cleared from the region of interest.

Colonoscopy, although valuable for assessing chronic and subacute bleeding, is not the examination of choice for acute rapid bleeding because the presence of fresh blood and clots prevents an adequate view of the mucosa.

 Caveat: Unstable patients with massive hemorrhage should have emergency surgery without any diagnostic studies.

Gastrointestinal Bleeding (Acute Upper)

Presenting Signs and Symptoms

Hematemesis, melena, ıematochezia
Blood in nasogastric aspirate

Common Causes

Peptic ulceration (duodenum, stomach, esophagus)
Gastric mucosal lesion (superficial erosions, stress ulcers)
Esophageal varices
Neoplasm
Mallory-Weiss tear

Approach to Diagnostic Imaging

▶ 1. **Endoscopy**
  - ▶ Procedure of choice that can permit precise visual identification of a lesion that is actively bleeding
  - ▶ Offers therapeutic options (electrocautery or laser cautery, mechanical clips, tissue adhesives, or injection of sclerosing agents for varices)
  - ▶ May be falsely negative if there is rapid bleeding, because large amounts of fresh blood and clots may obscure the underlying bleeding lesion

▶ 2. **Arteriography**
  - ▶ Indicated for patients with rapid bleeding (0.5–1 mL/min, but not if massive hemorrhage) in whom endoscopy is technically difficult
  - ▶ Demonstrates extravasation of contrast material or an angiodysplasia
  - ▶ Offers therapeutic options through transcatheter measures (embolization or infusion of vasoconstrictive agents); even if hemostasis fails or is only temporary, this technique generally allows time for vascular volume replacement to stabilize the patient before surgery

►3. **Upper gastrointestinal series**
  ► If bleeding is minimal or has stopped, this readily available, safe, and relatively inexpensive procedure is a good screening study for demonstrating an ulcer, neoplasm, or varices that *may* represent the bleeding site

---

Note: Introduction of barium into the gastrointestinal tract prevents the performance of endoscopy or arteriography until the barium has cleared from the region of interest.

 Caveat: Patients with massive hemorrhage whose conditions are unstable should have emergency surgery without any diagnostic studies.

Jaundice: Differentiation of Medical (Hepatocellular) from Surgical (Biliary Obstruction) Causes

Presenting Signs and Symptoms

Yellowing of skin and sclera
Abnormal liver enzymes
Dark urine and pale stools

Common Causes

Common duct stone
Pancreatic carcinoma
Cholangiocarcinoma
Primary hepatocellular dysfunction (alcoholism, hepatitis)

Approach to Diagnostic Imaging

▶ 1. **Ultrasound**
  ▶ Preferred screening technique for demonstrating dilated bile ducts (indicating biliary obstruction)
  ▶ May be equivocal or incomplete in obese patients or those with large amounts of intestinal gas

▶ 2. **Computed tomography**
  ▶ Highly accurate for showing dilated bile ducts as well as disease in adjacent structures (liver, porta hepatis, pancreas, adrenals, retroperitoneum)
  ▶ Not adversely affected by obesity or large amounts of intestinal gas

▶ 3. **Percutaneous transhepatic cholangiography (PTHC)**
  ▶ Invasive procedure of choice to define the precise site of obstruction in a dilated biliary system
  ▶ Superior to ERCP for diagnostic and therapeutic maneuvers (e.g., balloon dilatation of strictures, brush biopsies, stone removal, insertion of an endoprosthesis) that involve lesions above the porta hepatis (intrahepatic)
  ▶ Although it is generally safe, complications include sepsis, bile leakage with peritonitis, and bleeding

▶ 4. **Endoscopic retrograde cholangiopancreatography (ERCP)**
  ▶ Invasive procedure of choice if the bile ducts are not dilated (e.g., sclerosing cholangitis) and if the patient has abnormal bleeding parameters
  ▶ Permits therapeutic procedures such as sphincterotomy, stone extraction, brush biopsy of strictures, and insertion of an endoprosthesis

---

Note: Local experience often dictates the choice between PTHC and ERCP.

 Caveat: Although dilated bile ducts are virtually pathognomonic of extrahepatic biliary obstruction, normal bile ducts do not absolutely exclude this diagnosis because of the underlying disease process (e.g., sclerosing cholangitis) or because the obstruction may be recent or intermittent.

Nausea and Vomiting

Common Causes

Drug reaction (chemotherapeutic agents, CNS-active drugs, analgesics, cardiovascular drugs, hormones, antibiotics, diuretics, anti-asthmatics)

Gastrointestinal disorders

> Gastric outlet obstruction (peptic ulcer disease, gastric malignancy, extrinsic compression)
>
> Small bowel obstruction (adhesions, inflammatory bowel disease, neoplasm)
>
> Inflammatory conditions (gastroenteritis, peptic ulcer disease, cholecystitis, pancreatitis, Crohn's disease)
>
> Motility disorders (gastroparesis, irritable bowel syndrome, chronic intestinal pseudoobstruction, scleroderma)

Central nervous system disorders (stroke, neoplasm, labyrinthine disease, motion sickness, psychiatric disorders)

Metabolic conditions (pregnancy, uremia, hyperglycemia, hyperparathyroidism, metabolic acidosis, adrenal insufficiency)

Infectious disorders (hepatitis, meningitis, labyrinthitis)

Approach to Diagnostic Imaging

 Caveat: A detailed history, physical examination, and laboratory work-up should be performed initially. Appropriate imaging studies can then be ordered based on the probable clinical diagnosis.

SUSPECTED *GASTROINTESTINAL* CAUSE

▶ 1. **Plain abdominal radiograph**
   ▶ Inexpensive screening procedure for detecting a suspected gastric outlet or small bowel obstruction

▶ 2. **Computed tomography**
   ▶ Best study for detecting a suspected intraabdominal inflammatory process (and for further evaluation of small bowel obstruction demonstrated on plain films)

Peritonitis

Presenting Signs and Symptoms

Generalized abdominal tenderness with rigidity
Absence of bowel sounds
Fever
Vomiting

Common Causes

Perforation of a viscus
Trauma
Strangulating intestinal obstruction
Pancreatitis
Pelvic inflammatory disease
Vascular catastrophe (mesenteric thrombosis or embolus)
Ascites (spontaneous infection or peritoneo-systemic shunt)

Approach to Diagnostic Imaging

▶ 1. **Plain abdominal radiograph**
   - ▶ *Upright* films to demonstrate free air beneath the diaphragm indicating perforation of a viscus
   - ▶ If the patient cannot stand or sit, a *lateral decubitus* film (using a horizontal x-ray beam) with the patient's *left* side down may be used (any free air can be more easily detected over the soft-tissue-density liver on the right than when it is overlying luminal air in the stomach, small bowel, or splenic flexure on the left)
   - ▶ On *supine* films, look for the *double wall sign* (air outlining both the inner and outer walls of bowel loops) as well as free air outlining the normally invisible falciform and various pelvic ligaments

 Caveat: *NEVER* use barium in the presence of free air in the peritoneal cavity.

▶ 2. **Computed tomography**
   - ▶ Procedure of choice to detect loculated fluid collections, abscesses, and strangulating obstruction

Suspected Abdominal Abscess (No Localized Findings)

Presenting Signs and Symptoms

Spiking fever, leukocytosis, chills
Indolent course in immunosuppressed patient

Common Causes

Recent surgery or trauma
Alcoholism
Parenteral drug use
Chronic illness
Steroids, chemotherapy, immunosuppressive therapy

Approach to Diagnostic Imaging

► I. **Computed tomography**
  ► Preferred initial imaging procedure to detect, characterize, and determine the extent of an abdominal abscess
  ► Does not have the disadvantage of the substantial delay required with radionuclide scanning
  ► Limited value in patients with abrupt and extreme changes in density (metallic clips, residual barium) because of ''streak'' artifacts

▶ **2. Radionuclide scan (indium)**
- ▸ Can examine the entire abdomen simultaneously and detect multiple or extraabdominal sites of infection
- ▸ Scanning with indium is superior to gallium because normal accumulation of the latter in the liver, spleen, and colon can obscure an abscess; also, gallium (but not indium) can accumulate in lymphoma and other neoplasms

 Caveat: There is a substantial delay before diagnostic results can be obtained (at least 18–24 hours after radionuclide injection).

▶ **3. Ultrasound**
- ▸ Alternative to CT in very sick patients (who can suspend respiration only briefly)
- ▸ Multiplicity of scanning planes may be of value in assessing the precise anatomic relationships of a lesion
- ▸ Procedure of choice for children (uses no ionizing radiation)
- ▸ Because the examination requires close contact between the transducer and the skin, it may be difficult to perform on postsurgical patients with recent incisions, wound dressings, drains, superficial infections, or stomas

Hepatic Abscess

Presenting Signs and Symptoms

Subacute onset of fever, chills, nausea, anorexia, weight loss

Right upper quadrant pain

Hepatomegaly (acute onset suggests multiple abscesses from systemic bacteremia or biliary tract infection)

Common Causes

Ascending cholangitis in a partially or completely obstructed biliary tract

Portal bacteremia from an intraabdominal site (e.g., appendicitis, diverticulitis)

Systemic bacteremia (organisms reach liver through the hepatic artery)

Direct extension from adjacent extrabiliary site

Trauma

Approach to Diagnostic Imaging

▶ 1. **Computed tomography**
  ▶ Preferred study for detecting and characterizing an hepatic abscess

▶ 2. **Ultrasound**
  ▶ Alternative screening technique

Left Subphrenic Space

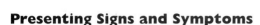

Presenting Signs and Symptoms

Left upper quadrant pain and tenderness
Fever and leukocytosis
History of surgery 3 to 6 weeks before onset

Common Causes

Surgery or trauma
Peritonitis (e.g., perforated viscus)
Spread from distant abdominal abscess

Approach to Diagnostic Imaging

▶ 1. **Computed tomography**
- ▶ Preferred screening study (negative CT scan excludes a left subphrenic abscess)
- ▶ Ultrasound is usually ineffective because of gas in the stomach, small bowel, or colon

▶ 2. **Radionuclide scan (indium or gallium)**
- ▶ Indicated if the CT scan is equivocal (not uncommon if there has been recent surgery or trauma), and it is impossible to differentiate an infected from a sterile collection (e.g., perisplenic hematoma)

 Caveat: Barium enema is contraindicated because retained barium within the bowel significantly delays the performance of more sensitive and specific studies such as CT and radionuclide scans.

Pancreas/Lesser Sac Abscess

Presenting Signs and Symptoms

Fever and abdominal pain arising 10 to 21 days after
acute pancreatitis
Nausea and vomiting
Abdominal mass
Leukocytosis
Increased serum amylase

Approach to Diagnostic Imaging

▶ 1. **Computed tomography**
  ▶ Preferred screening technique
  ▶ Ultrasound is generally ineffective because of the
    large amounts of intestinal gas related to the
    usually associated adynamic ileus

Perihepatic Abscess

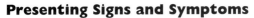

Presenting Signs and Symptoms

Right upper quadrant pain and tenderness
Fever and leukocytosis

Common Causes

Prior surgery or trauma

Approach to Diagnostic Imaging

▶ 1. **Plain abdominal radiograph**
  ▶ Can detect subtle perihepatic gas collections
  ▶ Localized ileus of the hepatic flexure and right pleural effusion are both suggestive but not diagnostic signs, since they may merely reflect nonspecific postoperative or post-traumatic changes

▶ 2. **Computed tomography**
  ▶ Preferred screening technique

▶ 3. **Ultrasound**
  ▶ Alternative screening technique

▶ 4. **Radionuclide scan (indium or gallium)**
  ▶ Examination of the entire abdomen and pelvis is indicated if an occult abscess is still suspected clinically despite negative ultrasound and CT studies
  ▶ Negative indium or gallium radionuclide scan effectively excludes an abscess

Pelvic Abscess

Presenting Signs and Symptoms

Lower abdominal pain and tenderness
Fever and leukocytosis
Palpable mass on vaginal or rectal examination

Common Causes

Acute appendicitis
Pelvic inflammatory disease
Colon diverticulitis

Approach to Diagnostic Imaging

▶ 1. **Ultrasound**
  ▸ Preferred screening technique
  ▸ Fluid-filled urinary bladder provides an excellent acoustic window for examining the supravesical and paravesical spaces

▶ 2. **Radionuclide scan**
  ▸ May be necessary to confirm the inflammatory nature of the lesion because the differential diagnosis of cystic masses is large

   Caveat: Indium is the preferred radionuclide because gallium normally accumulates in the sigmoid and rectum.

Renal/Perirenal Abscess

Presenting Signs and Symptoms

Acute onset of unilateral flank or abdominal pain and tenderness

Dysuria

Leukocytosis, fever, chills

Common Cause

Pyelonephritis (often associated with renal calculous disease, recent urologic surgery, or obstruction by malignancy)

Approach to Diagnostic Imaging

▶ 1. **Computed tomography**
  ▶ Preferred screening technique for detecting inflammatory and infectious renal disease
  ▶ May demonstrate thickening of Gerota's fascia, a subtle change that may be the first sign of a perirenal infection

▶ 2. **Ultrasound**
  ▶ Alternative screening technique that demonstrates a fluid-filled intrarenal or perirenal collection

Splenic Abscess

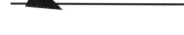

Presenting Signs and Symptoms

Subacute onset of left-sided pain (often pleuritic) in the flank, upper abdomen, or lower chest that may radiate to the left shoulder

Left upper quadrant tenderness

Splenomegaly

Leukocytosis and fever

Common Causes

Systemic bacteremia (e.g., endocarditis, salmonellosis)

Trauma (superinfection of hematoma)

Extension from contiguous infection (e.g., subphrenic abscess)

Approach to Diagnostic Imaging

▶ 1. **Computed tomography**
  - ▶ Preferred screening technique
  - ▶ Ultrasound is of less value because most of the spleen lies between the ribs and is largely hidden from the ultrasound beam

▶ 2. **Radionuclide scan (indium or gallium)**
  - ▶ Can specifically identify an intrasplenic mass as an abscess

Abdominal Mass
in a Neonate

Organ of Origin

Kidney

Gastrointestinal tract

Approach to Diagnostic Imaging

▶ 1. **Plain abdominal radiograph**
   ▶ To exclude obstruction of the gastrointestinal tract

▶ 2. **Ultrasound**
   ▶ Can detect intrinsic renal masses and hydrone-phrosis
   ▶ If ultrasound is normal, no further imaging is required
   ▶ If ultrasound detects a mass, further imaging depends on the anatomic location and sonographic characteristics of the lesion

Abdominal Mass in a Child

Organ of Origin

Kidney

Adrenal

Pelvic structure

Approach to Diagnostic Imaging

▶ 1. **Plain abdominal radiograph**
   - ▶ Can detect characteristic calcification associated with neuroblastoma (and its metastases)

▶ 2. **Ultrasound**
   - ▶ Best screening modality for detecting masses in the kidney, adrenal gland, or genital organs in a child (uses no ionizing radiation)
   - ▶ Can detect appendiceal abscesses or hepatobiliary lesions, the most common causes of gastrointestinal masses that develop after the neonatal period

▶ 3. **Excretory urography and voiding cystourethrography**
   - ▶ If ultrasound shows a cystic renal mass or severe hydronephrosis, these studies can evaluate kidney function, define the bladder anatomy, and confirm or exclude vesicoureteral reflux

▶ 4. **Computed tomography**
   - ▶ Indicated if ultrasound shows a solid mass suggestive of malignancy (to better define the anatomy as well as any local or metastatic spread)

Diffusely Enlarged Abdomen (No Discrete Mass)

Common Causes

Ascites
Lipodystrophy
Massive peritoneal/retroperitoneal tumor

Approach to Diagnostic Imaging

▶ I. **Computed tomography**
  ▶ Best modality for defining the organ of origin of any mass in the peritoneal or retroperitoneal compartments
  ▶ In patients with massive ascites, CT can suggest the cause of the peritoneal fluid by detecting masses, metastases, loculation, and the relative distribution of fluid in the lesser and greater sacs
  ▶ Adequate ultrasound examination is often prevented by gas contained within the stomach, small bowel, and colon

Epigastric Mass

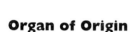

Organ of Origin

Liver
Spleen
Stomach
Duodenum
Pancreas

Approach to Diagnostic Imaging

▶ 1. **Computed tomography**
   ▸ Directly images the liver, spleen, gastric wall, and pancreas
   ▸ Adequate ultrasound examination is often prevented by gas contained within the stomach, small bowel, and colon

▶ 2. **Upper gastrointestinal series**
   ▸ If there is evidence of gastric outlet obstruction, it can evaluate for peptic ulcer or gastric malignancy

Hypogastric Mass

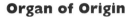

Organ of Origin

Bladder
Colon
Uterus
Ovary

Approach to Diagnostic Imaging

▶ 1. **Ultrasound**
   ▶ Preferred screening technique because most masses in this region are related to the pelvic organs

▶ 2. **Computed tomography**
   ▶ Indicated to better define the extent of the lesion if a solid mass is detected by ultrasound

▶ 3. **Barium enema**
   ▶ Indicated if the clinical examination suggests a gastrointestinal tumor as the underlying cause

Left Lower Quadrant Mass

Organ of Origin

Colon

Approach to Diagnostic Imaging

▶ 1. **Plain abdominal radiograph**
  ▶ Can demonstrate large bowel obstruction or fecal impaction

▶ 2. **Computed tomography**
  ▶ Preferred screening technique to detect and define the origin of a palpable mass or the extent of diverticulitis

▶ 3. **Barium enema**
  ▶ Can detect free or walled-off perforation or eccentric narrowing of the colonic lumen related to diverticulitis (the most likely clinical diagnosis)

 Caveat: If free perforation into the peritoneal cavity is suspected, *water-soluble* contrast must be used.

Left Upper Quadrant Mass

Organ of Origin

Spleen
Left lobe of the liver
Stomach (gastric outlet obstruction or tumor)
Splenic flexure of the colon
Pancreas
Left kidney
Left adrenal gland

Approach to Diagnostic Imaging

▶ 1. **Computed tomography**
- ▶ Directly images the spleen, liver, gastric wall, pancreas, left kidney, and left adrenal gland
- ▶ Adequate ultrasound examination is often precluded by gas contained within the stomach, small bowel, and colon

▶ 2. **Upper gastrointestinal series**
- ▶ If there is evidence of gastric outlet obstruction, it can evaluate for peptic ulcer or gastric malignancy

Midabdominal Mass

Organ of Origin

Superficial structures
Peritoneal structures
Retroperitoneal structures

Approach to Diagnostic Imaging

▶ 1. **Computed tomography**
  - ▶ Directly images the organs within all three compartments
  - ▶ Adequate ultrasound examination is often prevented by gas contained within the stomach, small bowel, and colon

▶ 2. **Ultrasound**
  - ▶ Initial modality of choice in an asthenic patient with a pulsating mass suggesting aortic aneurysm

Right Lower Quadrant Mass

Organ of Origin

Gastrointestinal tract
Abscess
Enlarged lymph nodes

Approach to Diagnostic Imaging

▶ 1. **Plain abdominal radiograph**
- ▶ Can exclude or confirm bowel obstruction, appendicolith, or fecal impaction

▶ 2. **Computed tomography**
- ▶ Can differentiate among such entities as inflammatory bowel disease, abscess, and enlarged lymph nodes

Right Upper Quadrant Mass

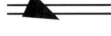

Organ of Origin

Right lobe of the liver
Gallbladder
Bile ducts
Right kidney
Right adrenal gland
Hepatic flexure of the colon
Duodenum

Imaging Approach

▶ **1. Ultrasound**
- ▶ High accuracy for detecting masses involving the gallbladder (acute cholecystitis, hydrops, carcinoma, Courvoisier gallbladder) and bile ducts, as well as diffuse and focal hepatic abnormalities
- ▶ Good screening test for detecting renal lesions and differentiating renal cysts from solid tumors or abscesses

▶ **2. Computed tomography**
- ▶ Indicated if there is bile duct dilatation and ultrasound fails to show an obstructing mass
- ▶ Indicated for confirmation and staging if ultrasound shows a solid renal mass
- ▶ Best modality for detecting adrenal masses (metastases, adenomas, carcinomas)

▶ **3. Barium enema or upper gastrointestinal series**
- ▶ Highest accuracy for detecting carcinoma of the hepatic flexure or the duodenum

Achalasia

Presenting Signs and Symptoms

Dysphagia for solids and liquids (typically in persons between 20 and 40 years old)

Nocturnal regurgitation of undigested food

Aspiration (and recurrent pneumonia)

Common Causes

Primary (idiopathic)

Malignancy (primary or metastatic)

Central and peripheral neuropathy

Cerebrovascular accident

Postvagotomy syndrome

Chagas disease

Approach to Diagnostic Imaging

▶ 1. **Plain chest radiograph**
   - ▶ Although not sensitive, plain chest radiographs may demonstrate such characteristic findings as an absent gastric air bubble and an esophageal air-fluid level

▶ 2. **Barium swallow**
   - ▶ Dilated esophagus with distal "beak" or "rat-tail" narrowing and an esophageal air-fluid level
   - ▶ Absence of the gastric air bubble

▶ 3. **Manometry**
   - ▶ Incomplete relaxation of the lower esophageal sphincter
   - ▶ Absent peristalsis in the smooth-muscle portion of the esophagus

Cancer of the Esophagus

Presenting Signs and Symptoms

Progressive dysphagia (first with solids, then liquids)
Pain (substernal or in the back due to local invasion)
Rapid weight loss
Pulmonary aspiration

Risk Factors

Ethanol abuse
Smoking
Lye ingestion and esophageal stricture
Radiation exposure
Head and neck cancer
Achalasia
Barrett's mucosa
Tylosis

Approach to Diagnostic Imaging

▶ 1. **Esophagram**
  ▶ Preferred screening examination that can detect superficial and early (small) tumors if the double-contrast technique is employed
  ▶ Cannot identify carcinoma *in situ*

▶ 2. **Esophagoscopy (with biopsy and cytology)**
  ▶ Most sensitive and specific test

Staging

▶ 1. **Computed tomography (chest/upper abdomen)**
  - ▶ Most effective staging procedure that can determine the potential surgical curability of an esophageal tumor in about 90% of patients
  - ▶ Accuracy of 97% for detecting tracheobronchial invasion and 94% for aortic and pericardial invasion
  - ▶ Demonstration of enlarged mediastinal or subdiaphragmatic lymph nodes is likely to represent involvement by metastatic tumor, although the absence of lymphadenopathy is an unreliable finding (since normal-sized nodes also may harbor metastases)

▶ 2. **Endoscopic ultrasound**
  - ▶ Superior to CT for evaluating the depth of tumor infiltration within the wall of the esophagus (local invasion) and lymph node involvement

---

Note: Ultrasound is not as effective as CT in assessing the extraesophageal spread of tumor, which relates directly to the duration of survival.

Diffuse Esophageal Spasm

Presenting Signs and Symptoms

Intermittent substernal chest pain

Dysphagia for both liquids and solids

Symptoms frequently aggravated by very hot or cold liquids

Approach to Diagnostic Imaging

▶ 1. **Barium swallow**
   - ▶ Corkscrew esophagus with pseudodiverticula

▶ 2. **Manometry**
   - ▶ Most sensitive and specific description of the spasms
   - ▶ High-amplitude esophageal contractions of long duration with repetitive occurrence

Esophageal Laceration (Mallory-Weiss Syndrome)

Presenting Signs and Symptoms

Repeated vomiting followed by hematemesis (especially in men over age 50 with history of alcohol abuse)

Approach to Diagnostic Imaging

▶ 1. **Endoscopy**
  ▶ Required to demonstrate the superficial lacerations or fissures near the esophagogastric junction (usually not seen on radiographic contrast studies)

Note: In rare cases, an esophagram shows contrast penetration into the wall of the esophagus.

Esophageal Perforation

Presenting Signs and Symptoms

Sudden epigastric pain radiating to the shoulder blades after vomiting, retching, or even hiccups (especially after heavy drinking)

Gravely ill appearance with pallor, sweating, tachycardia, and often shock

Common Causes

Boerhaave's syndrome
Penetrating trauma
Complication of endoscopy

Approach to Diagnostic Imaging

▶ 1. **Plain chest radiograph**

 ▶ Screening test to detect air dissecting within the mediastinum and soft tissues, often with pleural effusion or hydropneumothorax

▶ 2. **Barium swallow**

 ▶ May demonstrate extravasation through a transmural perforation

  Caveat: *Water-soluble* **contrast material must be used first (since barium cannot be cleared from the mediastinum); if no gross extravasation is shown, use barium (a better contrast agent) to exclude a small leak.**

▶ 3. **Computed tomography**

 ▶ Preferred study to define the extent of an inflammatory process in the mediastinum secondary to an esophageal perforation

Reflux Esophagitis

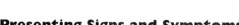

Presenting Signs and Symptoms

Heartburn

Dysphagia (due to stricture)

Upper gastrointestinal bleeding (due to esophageal ulceration)

Approach to Diagnostic Imaging

▶ 1. **Upper gastrointestinal series**
  - ▸ Frequent false negatives for gastroesophageal reflux and subtle esophagitis

▶ 2. **Endoscopy (with mucosal biopsy)**
  - ▸ Preferred study in the patient with active bleeding
  - ▸ Directly detects esophagitis and peptic strictures
  - ▸ May be normal in gastroesophageal reflux

Scleroderma

Presenting Signs and Symptoms

Often asymptomatic

Heartburn and dysphagia (due to reflux esophagitis secondary to incompetence of lower esophageal sphincter)

Approach to Diagnostic Imaging

▶ 1. **Barium swallow**
   ▶ Dilated esophagus with lack of peristalsis
   ▶ Widely patent distal esophagus (in the region of the lower esophageal sphincter)

> **Note:** The distal esophagus may be narrowed in chronic disease because of secondary reflux esophagitis.

▶ 2. **Manometry**
   ▶ Aperistalsis (due to atrophy of esophageal smooth muscle)
   ▶ Incompetent lower esophageal sphincter (leading to reflux esophagitis and stricture formation)

Varices
(Esophageal/Gastric)

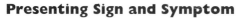

Presenting Sign and Symptom

Upper gastrointestinal bleeding

Common Causes

Cirrhosis
Obstruction of the splenic or portal vein (e.g., carcinoma of the pancreas)
Hepatic vein obstruction

Approach to Diagnostic Imaging

▶ 1. **Endoscopy**
  ▶ Procedure of choice for acute bleeding

▶ 2. **Barium swallow**
  ▶ Can demonstrate characteristic tortuous, beaded filling defects in the distal esophagus and gastric fundus

Interventive Radiologic Alternative

▶ 1. **Transjugular intrahepatic portosystemic shunt (TIPS)**
  ▶ Reported to be an effective and reliable means of lowering portal venous pressure, particularly in patients with acute variceal bleeding unresponsive to sclerotherapy and in patients with chronic variceal bleeding before liver transplantation

Cancer of the Stomach

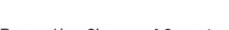

Presenting Signs and Symptoms

Progressive upper abdominal discomfort
Weight loss, anorexia, nausea, vomiting
Acute or chronic upper gastrointestinal bleeding
Early satiety

Risk Factors

Dietary habits (nitrates, smoked or heavily salted foods)
Atrophic gastritis (pernicious anemia)
Billroth II gastroenterostomy
Adenomatous gastric polyps

Approach to Diagnostic Imaging

▶ 1. **Double-contrast upper gastrointestinal series**
   - ▶ Preferred screening procedure
   - ▶ Requires meticulous technique to detect small, early lesions

▶ 2. **Endoscopy (with biopsy and cytology)**
   - ▶ Most sensitive and specific test (sensitivity of up to 98% if multiple biopsy specimens are taken from a suspicious lesion to decrease the risk of sampling error)
   - ▶ Much less accurate in detecting scirrhous lesions

Staging

▶ 1. **Computed tomography**
   - ▶ Most effective staging procedure for demonstrating the presence and extent of extragastric spread of tumor
   - ▶ More accurate in detecting distant lymphadenopathy than local lymph node enlargement

Peptic Ulcer Disease

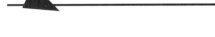

Presenting Signs and Symptoms

Burning epigastric pain (90–180 minutes after meals, often nocturnal, relieved by food)

Chronic, recurring course

Gastrointestinal bleeding (melena, hematemesis, hematochezia)

Gastric outlet obstruction (about 5%)

Acute abdomen (if free perforation)

Approach to Diagnostic Imaging

▶ **1. Upper gastrointestinal series**

  ▶ Signs of benignancy include a smooth ulcer mound with tapering edges, an edematous ulcer collar with overhanging mucosal edge, projection of the ulcer beyond the expected lumen, and thin radiating folds extending into the crater

  ▶ Size, depth, number, and location of the ulcer are of no diagnostic value in differentiating benign from malignant (except for ulcers in the cardia, which are virtually always malignant)

▶ **2. Endoscopy**

  ▶ May be preferable for suspected gastric ulcer, since biopsy can be performed to exclude malignancy (1% of radiographically benign-appearing ulcers prove to be malignant)

  ▶ More reliable for detecting acute ulcer craters in a scarred duodenum

  ▶ Fails to detect 5–10% of peptic ulcers

   Caveat: Once the diagnosis of benign peptic disease has been made, recurrences should be treated symptomatically; there is *no* need to repeat an imaging procedure with each recurrence.

Zollinger-Ellison Syndrome

Presenting Signs and Symptoms

Refractory peptic ulcer disease (after medical therapy or surgery)

Gastric hypersecretion

Diarrhea

Substantially elevated serum gastrin

Common Cause

Gastrinoma (usually of the pancreas)

Approach to Diagnostic Imaging

▶ 1. **Computed tomography**
   - ▶ Preferred study for detecting the underlying pancreatic tumor, which typically is small, often multiple, and intensely enhancing

▶ 2. **Upper gastrointestinal series**
   - ▶ May show characteristic pattern of markedly thickened gastric folds and ulcers distal to the duodenal bulb (seen in about half the cases)

Gastroenteritis

Presenting Signs and Symptoms

Anorexia, nausea, vomiting
Diarrhea of variable severity
Abdominal discomfort
Low-grade fever
Travel history

Common Causes

Bacterial, viral, or parasitic infection
Enterotoxins (bacterial)
Chemical toxins (mushrooms, shellfish, contaminated
food)
Food allergies

Approach to Diagnostic Imaging

No imaging studies are required unless examinations of
stool specimens and stool cultures are negative and the
symptoms persist

Small Bowel Obstruction

Presenting Signs and Symptoms

Crampy abdominal pain and bloating
Nausea and vomiting
Abdominal tenderness and peritoneal signs
Abdominal distension
Increased high-pitched bowel sounds

Common Causes

Adhesions
Hernia
Tumor
Intussusception
Extrinsic mass

Approach to Diagnostic Imaging

▶ 1. **Plain abdominal radiograph**
   ▶ Change in caliber of air-filled bowel (dilated proximally; collapsed distally)
   ▶ String-of-beads sign on upright films

► **2. Computed tomography (optional)**

> ► Only required to confirm an obstruction if plain films are equivocal or if it is necessary to show the precise site of obstruction

> ► Much more accurate than small bowel follow through with oral contrast agent for demonstrating the underlying cause of the obstruction

 Caveat: If CT scan is inconclusive and an oral contrast examination is needed to confirm an obstruction, use barium and *NOT* water-soluble agents for small bowel follow through (hyperosmolar contrast draws fluid into the bowel, diluting the opaque material and making it difficult to show the site of obstruction clearly). Before giving barium by mouth, it is necessary to exclude a large bowel obstruction (use water-soluble contrast).

Antibiotic-Associated Colitis

Presenting Signs and Symptoms

Range from transient mild diarrhea to a severe colitis that develops during a course of antibiotic therapy or up to 6 weeks after treatment has ceased

Common Causes

Due to toxin-producing strains of *C. difficile* (especially after clindamycin, ampicillin, cephalosporins, aminoglycosides)

Approach to Diagnostic Imaging

► 1. **Sigmoidoscopy**
  ► Directly shows characteristic pseudomembranes

► 2. **Computed tomography**
  ► Demonstrates mural thickening of a hypodense colon wall
  ► Because symptoms may be misleading, CT may suggest the correct diagnosis before it is suspected clinically

 Caveat: Although barium enema may show the extent of mucosal abnormalities, it is *contraindicated* in active or severe cases because of the risk of perforation.

Appendicitis

Presenting Signs and Symptoms

Sudden onset of epigastric or periumbilical pain that shifts to the right lower quadrant

Rebound tenderness

Low-grade fever and leukocytosis

Approach to Diagnostic Imaging

▶ 1. **Plain abdominal radiograph**
  ▶ Although of low sensitivity and specificity, plain abdominal radiographs may detect a calcified appendicolith (about 15%) that is strongly suggestive of impending perforation

▶ 2. **Ultrasound**
  ▶ High sensitivity and specificity without need for ionizing radiation (especially in children and women during childbearing years)
  ▶ Disadvantages include high operator-dependence and limitations due to obesity and large amounts of intestinal gas

▶ 3. **Computed tomography**
  ▶ Imaging method of choice for suspected periappendiceal abscess
  ▶ Highly accurate for showing unrelated intraabdominal disease that may mimic appendicitis and explain the patient's clinical presentation
  ▶ Can be used to guide percutaneous abscess drainage
  ▶ Detects appendicolith in about 30% of cases

 Caveat: Normal CT scan does not unequivocally exclude appendicitis, because mild forms without periappendiceal disease may escape detection.

Cancer of the Colon

Presenting Signs and Symptoms

Bright red rectal bleeding, altered bowel habits, abdominal or back pain (left-sided lesions)

Iron deficiency anemia, occult blood in the stool, weight loss (right-sided lesions)

Risk Factors

Diet (low in fiber, high in animal fat)
Personal or family history of colorectal polyps
Familial polyposis syndrome
Family history of colorectal cancer
Ulcerative colitis
Crohn's colitis
Hypercholesterolemia

Approach to Diagnostic Imaging

▶ 1. **Double-contrast barium enema**
  - ▶ Preferred screening procedure
  - ▶ Requires meticulous technique to detect small, early lesions

▶ 2. **Colonoscopy/flexible sigmoidoscopy**
  - ▶ Slightly more sensitive and specific than barium enema, but associated with considerably higher cost and complications
  - ▶ Blind spots behind folds or around the flexures

Staging

► **1. Computed tomography**
- ► Most effective staging procedure for demonstrating the presence and extent of extracolonic spread of tumor

► **2. Transrectal ultrasound**
- ► Most accurate imaging method for staging local rectal cancer (can assess the depth of invasion within the bowel wall and suggest the presence of tumor in adjacent lymph nodes that are of normal size)

Crohn's Disease

Presenting Signs and Symptoms

Abdominal pain

Fever

Anorexia and weight loss

Diarrhea (often without blood)

Fatigue

Right lower quadrant mass or fullness

Anorectal fissures, fistulas, abscesses (may be acute ileitis mimicking appendicitis or obstruction)

Complications include bowel obstruction, internal fistulas, and bile salt malabsorption leading to gallstones or oxalate kidney stones

Approach to Diagnostic Imaging

▶ **1. Barium enema**

  ▶ Demonstrates involvement of the terminal ileum and variable amounts of colon and more proximal small bowel disease characterized by nodularity and thickening of folds, aphthous ulcers, narrowing and rigidity, cobblestoning, string sign, skip areas, and fistulas

▶ **2. Small bowel examination**

  ▶ Required if the terminal ileum is not visualized because of an inability to reflux barium through a competent ileocecal valve

▶ **3. Computed tomography**

  ▶ In addition to showing thickening of the bowel wall, this is the best imaging modality for demonstrating mesenteric and extraintestinal extent of disease and abscess formation

Ulcerative Colitis

Presenting Signs and Symptoms

Bloody diarrhea

Mucus in the stools

Abdominal pain (spectrum of severity ranging from mild lower abdominal cramping to severe peritoneal signs)

Fever

Complications (toxic megacolon, colon perforation, hemorrhage, increased risk of cancer)

Approach to Diagnostic Imaging

▶ 1. **Sigmoidoscopy**
   ▶ Direct and immediate indication of the activity of the disease process

▶ 2. **Plain abdominal radiograph**
   ▶ Must exclude toxic megacolon *before* attempting a barium enema
   ▶ Distal extent of formed fecal residue gives a good indication (although not absolute) of the proximal extent of the colitis (may overestimate, but does not underestimate the extent of disease)

▶ 3. **Barium enema or colonoscopy**
   ▶ To determine the full extent of the disease and to detect the development of malignancy in patients with chronic disease

Diverticulitis

Presenting Signs and Symptoms

Abdominal pain and tenderness (typically left lower quadrant)

Fever and leukocytosis

Altered bowel habits

Approach to Diagnostic Imaging

▶ 1. **Computed tomography**
- ▶ Demonstrates pericolonic fluid or a gas collection (abscess), usually with nonspecific thickening of the colon wall, narrowing of the colon lumen, and inflammatory stranding in adjacent fat
- ▶ Can be used to guide percutaneous abscess drainage

▶ 2. **Barium enema**
- ▶ May demonstrate extravasation of contrast through a diverticular perforation *or* a pericolic soft-tissue mass (walled-off perforation) causing eccentric narrowing of the colon

 Caveat: If free perforation into the peritoneal cavity is suspected, *water-soluble* contrast must be used.

Note: Plain abdominal radiographs are *not* needed unless there are peritoneal signs suggesting free perforation.

Diverticulosis

Presenting Signs and Symptoms

Often asymptomatic
Unexplained lower gastrointestinal bleeding
Recurrent left lower quadrant pain
Alternating constipation and diarrhea

Approach to Diagnostic Imaging

▶ 1. Barium enema
- ▶ Contrast-filled outpouchings from the colon without evidence of extravasation or mass effect

 Caveat: It can be extremely difficult to exclude a polyp or carcinoma in a segment of colon that is severely involved by diverticular disease.

Hemorrhoids

Presenting Signs and Symptoms

Bleeding (typically after defecation and noted on the toilet tissue)

Pain (if ulcerated, thrombosed, or strangulated)

Protrusion (may regress spontaneously or be reduced manually)

Approach to Diagnostic Imaging

There is *no* indication for any imaging procedure. A barium enema examination should only be performed if there is clinical evidence of a more serious cause of rectal bleeding (hemorrhoidal bleeding rarely leads to anemia or an acute exsanguinating hemorrhage).

Irritable Bowel Syndrome

Presenting Signs and Symptoms

Symptoms triggered by stress or ingestion of foods
Pasty, ribbon-like, or pencil-thin stools
Mucus (not blood) in the stools
Onset often before age 30 (especially in women)

Common Variants

Spastic colon (chronic abdominal pain and constipation)
Alternating constipation and diarrhea
Chronic painless diarrhea

Approach to Diagnostic Imaging

▶ I. **Barium enema**
  ▶ Primarily performed to exclude inflammatory bowel disease or malignancy

Large Bowel Obstruction

Presenting Signs and Symptoms

Gradually increasing constipation leading to obstipation and abdominal distension

Lower abdominal cramps unproductive of feces

Vomiting (if incompetent ileocecal valve)

Common Causes

Malignant tumor

Inflammatory stricture (e.g., diverticulitis)

Volvulus

Hernia

Extrinsic lesion

Approach to Diagnostic Imaging

▶ I. **Plain abdominal radiograph**

- ▶ Change in caliber of gas-filled colon at the site of obstruction
- ▶ Lateral decubitus view (right-side down) can allow gas to rise into the sigmoid and rectum and differentiate between colonic ileus (rectum/sigmoid distended) and mechanical obstruction (rectum/sigmoid remain collapsed)

▶ 2. **Barium enema**
  ▶ Shows site and character of the obstruction

Notes: In patients with *acute* obstruction, *water-soluble* contrast material should be used (due to the danger of barium inspissation proximal to a colonic obstruction; if there is an adynamic ileus, retained barium will remain for a prolonged period and interfere with other imaging studies).

In patients with intussusception or volvulus, a barium enema may be therapeutic as well as diagnostic.

If endoscopy is to be performed, it should *precede* the barium enema.

▶ 3. **Computed tomography**
  ▶ Especially valuable in patients without a history of surgery who have systemic signs suggesting infection, bowel infarction, or an associated palpable mass
  ▶ Can demonstrate diverticulitis or appendicitis as the cause of an obstruction

Note: Some radiologists recommend CT as the initial study (instead of barium enema) as a more direct means for establishing the diagnosis of large bowel obstruction.

Cholecystitis (Acute)

Presenting Signs and Symptoms

Acute colicky right upper quadrant pain and tenderness
Fever
Nausea and vomiting
Mild jaundice (occasionally)

Laboratory Findings

Mild leukocytosis
Mild elevation of serum bilirubin, alkaline phosphatase,
serum glutamic oxaloacetic transaminase

Approach to Diagnostic Imaging

▶ 1. **Cholescintigraphy (technetium-IDA derivatives)**
  ▶ Visualized gallbladder *excludes* acute cholecystitis
   (95% specificity) by indicating patency of the
   cystic duct
  ▶ Nonvisualized gallbladder after 4 hours strongly
   suggests acute cholecystitis (98% sensitivity) if
   the patient is not a chronic alcoholic or undergoing total parenteral nutrition

Note: By using morphine augmentation, the time required to perform the radionuclide study is reduced
to 1.5 hours.

▶ **2. Ultrasound**
  ▸ May demonstrate gallstones, thickening of the gall-
    bladder wall, pericholecystic fluid, and point
    tenderness directly over the gallbladder (sono-
    graphic Murphy's sign)
  ▸ Permits detection of abnormalities of the liver, pan-
    creas, or kidneys that may produce a clinical ap-
    pearance mimicking acute cholecystitis (only
    about one-third of patients with symptoms of
    acute cholecystitis actually have that condition)
  ▸ Indicated if there is strong clinical evidence of acal-
    culous nonobstructing acute cholecystitis in the
    face of a negative cholescintigram

   Caveat: Do *not* order oral cholecystogra-
  phy (low sensitivity).

Cholecystitis (Chronic)

Presenting Signs and Symptoms

Recurrent right upper quadrant pain and biliary colic

Approach to Diagnostic Imaging

► 1. **Ultrasound**
- ► Preferred screening technique
- ► Demonstrates high-amplitude echo in the gallbladder lumen (reflecting from the surface of a gallstone) or in the gallbladder fossa (if the lumen is completely filled with calculi) associated with posterior acoustic shadowing

► 2. **Oral cholecystogram**
- ► Only indicated if ultrasound is negative or nondiagnostic in the face of strong clinical evidence of chronic cholecystitis
- ► Disadvantages include the need for a functioning gallbladder and serum bilirubin less than 3 mg/dL

 Caveat: Plain abdominal radiographs are of limited value, since only about 20% of gallstones are radiopaque.

Fatty Liver

Presenting Signs and Symptoms

Asymptomatic hepatomegaly

Possible right upper quadrant pain, tenderness, or jaundice

Common Causes

Cirrhosis

Chemicals/drugs (e.g., alcohol, steroids, tetracyclines, carbon tetrachloride, methotrexate)

Obesity

Malnutrition

Hyperalimentation

Cystic fibrosis

Approach to Diagnostic Imaging

▶ I. **Computed tomography**

    ▶ Noncontrast scans demonstrate diffuse low attenuation of the liver parenchyma (lower than that of the spleen)

    ▶ Focal fatty infiltration may simulate a liver tumor (although vessels typically run their normal course through the area of involvement)

Hemangioma of the Liver

Presenting Signs and Symptoms

Asymptomatic and discovered incidentally on ultrasound, CT, or MRI

Approach to Diagnostic Imaging

▶ I. **Ultrasound, computed tomography, magnetic resonance imaging, or radionuclide scan**

  ▶ Ultrasound may show a typically well-defined, hyperechoic mass

  ▶ CT may demonstrate a low-attenuation mass with well-defined borders on nonenhanced scans; after contrast injection, there may be characteristic filling in of the lesion in a centripetal fashion (entire mass becomes isointense)

  ▶ MRI may show marked hyperintensity of the mass on T2-weighted images with an enhancement pattern similar to that of CT

  ▶ Radionuclide scans using tagged red blood cells shows prolonged activity within the lesion on delayed images (preferred imaging study if the lesion is >3 cm)

Notes: If the lesion has a *characteristic* appearance, it should be left alone with no further imaging studies.

If the patient has a known malignancy, abnormal liver function tests, or symptoms, *more than one* imaging study should be performed.

Hepatocellular Carcinoma (Hepatoma)

Presenting Signs and Symptoms

Right upper quadrant pain
Tender hepatomegaly
Unexplained deterioration in a previously stable patient
 with cirrhosis
Weight loss
Fever (may simulate infection)
Elevated serum α-fetoprotein (in 90%)

Risk Factors

Chronic hepatitis B infection
Cirrhosis (especially alcohol-induced)
Hemochromatosis
Thorotrast (radiographic contrast agent used from about
 1940–1960)

Approach to Diagnostic Imaging

▶ 1. **Computed tomography**
  ▸ Preferred screening technique for demonstrating
   any of the three major patterns (diffuse infiltrative, solitary massive, and multinodular)

▶ 2. **Ultrasound**
  ▸ Used in high-prevalence areas (e.g., Japan) for
   screening of chronic hepatitis B virus carriers

▶ 3. **Magnetic resonance imaging**
  ▸ May permit a specific diagnosis of hepatocellular
   carcinoma by demonstrating (1) characteristic
   capsule of compressed liver or scar tissue, (2) accumulation of fat within the tumor, and (3) propensity of tumor spread into the hepatic and
   portal veins

Liver Metastases

Presenting Signs and Symptoms
Usually asymptomatic
May have nonspecific weight loss, anorexia, fever, weakness
Hepatomegaly (hard and often tender)
Ascites
Jaundice

Common Primary Tumors
Gastrointestinal tract (colon, pancreas, stomach)
Lung
Breast
Lymphoma
Melanoma

Approach to Diagnostic Imaging
► **1. Computed tomography**
  ► Sensitive screening technique that is preferred to MRI if there is also a need to assess possible metastases in the adrenal glands, retroperitoneum, and other abdominal organs
  ► Permits fine-needle aspiration biopsy for cytology to provide a definitive diagnosis

► **2. Magnetic resonance imaging**
  ► Sensitive technique for detecting liver metastases; generally is indicated in patients who cannot receive intravenous iodinated contrast or who are being considered for partial hepatectomy

► **3. Ultrasound**
  ► Although less sensitive than MRI or CT, ultrasound is rapid and inexpensive and reliably identifies the majority of patients with hepatic metastases

 Caveat: Radionuclide scanning is less sensitive than other methods for detecting liver metastases and thus is *not* indicated for routine screening.

Portal Hypertension

Presenting Signs and Symptoms

Bleeding esophageal varices
Ascites and edema
Encephalopathy
Nonspecific constitutional symptoms of fatigue, lethargy, anorexia

Common Causes

Cirrhosis
Obstruction of the extrahepatic portal vein (e.g., carcinoma of the pancreas)
Hepatic vein obstruction

Approach to Diagnostic Imaging

▶ 1. **Color and duplex Doppler**
  ▸ Demonstrates patency and the direction of blood flow in the hepatic veins, portal veins, and collateral venous channels

▶ 2. **Computed tomography**
  ▸ Documents the presence of venous collaterals in the mesentery and retroperitoneum
  ▸ Can better define the cause of extrahepatic portal vein thrombosis and any propagation into the liver

▶ 3. **Magnetic resonance angiography**
  ▸ Indicated if intravenous contrast material may not be given or if the CT scan is inconclusive

Pancreatitis (Acute)

Presenting Signs and Symptoms

Steady, boring midepigastric pain radiating straight through to the back

Elevated serum amylase and lipase

Common Causes

Biliary tract disease (e.g., stones)

Alcoholism

Drugs

Infection (e.g., mumps)

Hyperlipidemia

ERCP

Neoplasm

Surgery or trauma

Approach to Diagnostic Imaging

▶ 1. **Computed tomography**
  - ▶ Imaging procedure of choice for demonstrating focal or diffuse enlargement of the gland and indistinctness of its margins
  - ▶ Superior to ultrasound for showing extrapancreatic spread of inflammation and edema and for detecting gas within a pancreatic fluid collection (highly suggestive of abscess)
  - ▶ Can also be used to suggest the prognosis

▶**2. Ultrasound**
  ▶ In addition to demonstrating symmetric enlargement of a relatively sonolucent gland, ultrasound may show cholelithiasis, an important underlying cause of acute pancreatitis
  ▶ Frequent occurrence of adynamic ileus with excessive intestinal gas may prevent adequate visualization of the gland
  ▶ Useful for follow-up of specific abnormalities (such as fluid collections)

 Caveat: Although plain abdominal radiographs are abnormal in 50% of patients, they usually show only generalized or localized ileus that is *not specific* for pancreatitis.

Pancreatitis (Chronic)

Presenting Signs and Symptoms

Midepigastric pain

Weight loss, steatorrhea, and other signs and symptoms of malabsorption

Common Causes

Alcoholism

Hereditary pancreatitis

Hyperparathyroidism

Obstruction of main pancreatic duct (stricture, stones, cancer)

Approach to Diagnostic Imaging

▶ 1. **Plain abdominal radiograph**
   - ▶ Demonstrates virtually pathognomonic pancreatic calcifications in 30–60% of cases

▶ 2. **Computed tomography or ultrasound**
   - ▶ Shows enlargement or atrophy of the gland, dilatation of the pancreatic duct, and pseudocyst formation
   - ▶ CT is more accurate in demonstrating the focal superimposition of a malignant mass and is not adversely affected by the large amounts of intestinal gas that may accompany an acute exacerbation of inflammatory disease

▶ 3. **Endoscopic retrograde cholangiopancreatography (ERCP)**
   - ▶ Shows irregular dilatation of the main pancreatic duct and pruning of its branches

Cancer of the Pancreas

Presenting Signs and Symptoms

Abdominal and back pain
Weight loss and anorexia
Painless jaundice
Enlarged, palpable gallbladder (Courvoisier's sign)

Approach to Diagnostic Imaging

▶ 1. **Computed tomography**
- ▶ Shows a mass with (or without) obstructive dilatation of the pancreatic or bile duct or both
- ▶ Most effective modality for demonstrating lesions in the tail and for defining the extent of spread of tumor (may prevent needless surgery in patients with nonresectable lesions)

▶ 2. **Ultrasound**
- ▶ Useful screening test (shows abnormalities in about 75% of patients) but may fail to detect small lesions in the body and tail

▶ 3. **Endoscopic retrograde cholangiopancreatography (ERCP)**
- ▶ Most sensitive test for tumors of the pancreatic head (deformity/stricture of the bile duct)
- ▶ Indicated if clinical suspicion remains high in the face of normal CT and ultrasound examinations

Interventive Radiologic Alternatives

▶ 1. **Percutaneous fine-needle aspiration (under CT or ultrasound guidance)**
- ▶ Often provides a precise histologic diagnosis

▶ 2. **Percutaneous stent placement for biliary drainage**
- ▶ May be performed using either ERCP or PTHC

Trauma
(Blunt Abdominal)

Approach to Diagnostic Imaging

▶ **1. Plain abdominal and chest radiographs**
- ▶ Although neither sensitive nor specific, these inexpensive and rapidly available studies can direct attention to specific organ injuries
  - ▶ **Spleen**
    - ▶ Fracture of lower left ribs
    - ▶ Elevation of left hemidiaphragm
    - ▶ Left pleural effusion
    - ▶ Displacement of gastric air bubble
    - ▶ Irregular splenic outline
  - ▶ **Liver**
    - ▶ Fractures of right lower ribs
    - ▶ Displacement of hepatic flexure
    - ▶ Irregular/enlarged hepatic outline
  - ▶ **Retroperitoneum**
    - ▶ Loss of psoas or renal shadow
    - ▶ Free retroperitoneal gas
    - ▶ Fracture of lumbar transverse process
  - ▶ **Diaphragm**
    - ▶ Herniation of abdominal contents into chest
    - ▶ Abnormal position of nasogastric tube
    - ▶ Elevation and loss of definition of hemidiaphragm
    - ▶ Nonspecific pleural effusion and atelectasis

▶ **2. Computed tomography**
- ▶ Highest sensitivity and specificity for detecting injuries to the liver, spleen, kidneys, and retroperitoneum

▶ 3. **Radionuclide scan or ultrasound**
  ▸ Only indicated if CT examination of the liver and spleen is ambiguous because of surgical clip artifacts or motion (or if an allergy to intravenous contrast precludes an enhanced CT study)

▶ 4. **Arteriography**
  ▸ Only indicated if both CT and radionuclide scan are equivocal (especially valuable as both a diagnostic and therapeutic tool in patients with pelvic ring disruption who have evidence of severe bleeding)

 Caveat: **Diagnostic peritoneal lavage, although traditionally the generally accepted standard for the diagnosis of possible abdominal injury, has been replaced in most centers by CT. Diagnostic peritoneal lavage can yield false-negative results in injuries to retroperitoneal structures (kidneys, pancreas, duodenum) or the diaphragm. In addition, a positive peritoneal lavage occurs in up to 25% of patients with trivial injuries that do not require laparotomy and may occur in patients with pelvic fractures or as a result of a traumatic peritoneal tap.**

URINARY

N. Reed Dunnick

▶ SIGNS AND SYMPTOMS

Dysuria
Hematuria
  Painless
  Painful

Renal Failure
  Acute
  Chronic

▶ DISORDERS

Kidney
Inflammatory
Abscess
  Renal
  Perinephric (Perirenal)
  Pyelonephritis
  Acute
  Chronic
  Pyonephrosis
Urinary Tract Infection
  Infant
  Female Child
  Male Child

  Older Child/Teenager
  Adult

Mass
Renal Mass
Renal Cyst
Cancer (Hypernephroma)
Medullary Cystic Disease
Multicystic Dysplastic
    Kidney
Polycystic Kidney Disease
  Adult
  Childhood

Vascular
Atheroembolic Renal
Disease
Nephrosclerosis
(Malignant)
Renal Cortical Necrosis
Renal Infarction
Renal Vein Thrombosis
Renovascular
Hypertension

Trauma
Bladder
Renal
Blunt
Penetrating
Urethral

Bladder
Cancer
Neurogenic Bladder
Outlet Obstruction

Adrenal
Addison's Disease
Adrenal Virilism
(Adrenogenital
Syndrome)
Aldosteronism (Conn's
Syndrome)

Other
Glomerulonephritis
Acute
Chronic
Hydronephrosis
Medullary Sponge Kidney
Nephrocalcinosis
Nephrolithiasis (Urinary
Calculi)
Tubulointerstitial
Nephritis
Acute Tubular
Necrosis
Chronic

Cystitis
Urethritis (Gonococcal)

Cushing's Syndrome
Metastases
Pheochromocytoma

Dysuria

Common Causes

Urethritis (infection, catheters)
Cystitis (infection, radiation, chemicals, catheters, stones)
Prostatitis
Bladder tumor
Functional bladder syndrome

Approach to Diagnostic Imaging

 Caveat: In most cases, the cause of dysuria is evident from clinical examination and urinalysis, and no imaging procedures are necessary.

▶ I. **Excretory urography or voiding cystourethrography**
- ▶ Can demonstrate the diffuse irregular thickening of the bladder wall in inflammatory disease as well as a lucent filling defect resulting from a bladder stone or tumor

Hematuria (Painless)

Common Causes

Neoplasm (kidney, ureter, bladder, urethra)
Glomerulonephritis
Vascular abnormality (aneurysm, malformation, arterial or venous occlusion)
Papillary necrosis
Urolithiasis

Approach to Diagnostic Imaging

▶ 1. **Ultrasound**
    ▶ Relatively efficient imaging technique for detecting neoplastic renal masses and vascular anomalies

▶ 2. **Excretory urography**
    ▶ Excellent for detecting stones and papillary necrosis

     Caveat: Cannot exclude bladder or urethral pathology

▶ 3. **Cystoscopy**
    ▶ Required in any adult with unexplained hematuria because a normal ultrasound examination (and excretory urography) does not exclude a bladder tumor or cystitis

▶ 4. **Computed tomography**
    ▶ More sensitive than ultrasound or excretory urography for detecting renal masses

Hematuria (Painful)

Common Causes

Ureteral calculus, trauma, infection (especially cystitis or urethritis)

Approach to Diagnostic Imaging

▶ I. **Excretory urography**
  ▶ Preferred screening procedure that provides a broad range of morphologic and functional information concerning all portions of the urinary tract
  ▶ Can define the site of an impacted ureteral stone and the degree of resulting ureteral obstruction as well as any posttraumatic extravasation of contrast material from the urinary tract

---

Note: If there is complete ureteral obstruction, the excretory urogram may show nonvisualization of the ipsilateral kidney or a prolonged nephrogram with lack of filling of the ureter so that it may be impossible to determine the site of the impacted stone.

► **2. Ultrasound**
  - ► Can demonstrate the presence and degree of ureteral dilatation proximal to an impacted stone
  - ► In patients with a nonopaque, completely obstructing stone causing loss of ipsilateral kidney function, ultrasound can demonstrate the stone as an echogenic focus with acoustic shadowing
  - ► Ureteral stones may be obscured by bowel gas

► **3. Computed tomography**
  - ► An unenhanced scan can detect even poorly opaque stones (such as uric acid calculi)
  - ► Either unenhanced CT or ultrasound may be used in patients in whom the use of intravascular contrast media is contraindicated

Renal Failure (Acute)

Presenting Signs and Symptoms

Rapid, steadily increasing azotemia, with or without oliguria

Common Causes

PRERENAL

Hypovolemia (diarrhea, vomiting, hemorrhage, overdiuresis, pancreatitis, peritonitis)

Vasodilatation (sepsis, drugs, anaphylaxis)

Cardiac (congestive heart failure, myocardial infarction, cardiac tamponade)

Renal hypoperfusion (renal artery obstruction)

RENAL

Acute tubular injury (ischemia, toxins, hemoglobinuria, myoglobinuria, radiocontrast agents)

Acute glomerulonephritis

Acute tubular nephritis (drug reaction, pyelonephritis, papillary necrosis)

Precipitation of substances within the kidney (calcium, urates, myeloma protein)

Arterial or venous obstruction

Disseminated intravascular coagulopathy with cortical necrosis

POSTRENAL

Calculi

Prostatism

Neoplasm (bladder, pelvic, retroperitoneal)

Retroperitoneal fibrosis

Urethral or bladder neck obstruction

Approach to Diagnostic Imaging

▶ **1. Ultrasound**

 ▸ Screening procedure of choice to assess renal size, identify renal parenchymal disease (diffuse increase in echogenicity with loss of corticomedullary differentiation), and exclude hydronephrosis (postrenal cause)

> **Note:** In patients with acute renal failure and *large* (>12 cm) or normal-sized kidneys, biopsy is often required for definitive diagnosis of renal parenchymal disease; patients with *small* (<9 cm) kidneys usually have irreversible end-stage renal disease and do not benefit from biopsy.

 ▸ If a vascular cause is suggested clinically, color Doppler studies may demonstrate patency or occlusion of the renal artery or vein. If this is unsuccessful, radionuclide renal scan or magnetic resonance imaging can show these vessels.

 Caveat: Although arteriography and venography are more definitive tests for vascular occlusion, some physicians prefer not to use radiographic contrast agents in the patient with acute renal failure.

Renal Failure (Chronic)

Presenting Signs and Symptoms

Irreversible loss of renal function (uremia)

Neuromuscular (peripheral neuropathy, muscle cramps, convulsions, encephalopathy)

Gastrointestinal (anorexia, nausea and vomiting, peptic ulcer, unpleasant taste in the mouth)

Cardiopulmonary (congestive heart failure, hypertension, pericarditis, pleural effusion)

Skin (uremic frost, pruritus)

Secondary hyperparathyroidism

Common Causes

Diabetic nephropathy

Hypertension

Glomerulonephritis

Polycystic kidney disease (autosomal dominant)

Approach to Diagnostic Imaging

▶ I. **Ultrasound**

> ▶ Screening procedure of choice that can assess kidney size (usually small kidneys in chronic renal failure) as well as detect hydronephrosis secondary to obstruction (especially in patients with risk factors such as known or suspected pelvic malignancy, renal calculus disease, or bladder outlet obstruction)

Renal Abscess

Presenting Signs and Symptoms

Fever, leukocytosis, and flank pain

Frequently a history of prior antibiotic therapy with relapse on cessation

Approach to Diagnostic Imaging

▶ **1. Computed tomography**

  ▸ Preferred study for demonstrating the thick-walled, low-attenuation mass within the kidney that may extend to the perirenal space (usually thickening of Gerota's fascia and strands of increased density in the adjacent fat)

  ▸ Gas within the mass is virtually pathognomonic of renal abscess

   Caveat: There is *no* indication for excretory urography in the patient with a suspected renal abscess.

▶ **2. Ultrasound**

  ▸ Alternative method for demonstrating a renal or perinephric abscess, but less sensitive than CT

▶ **3. Interventive radiology**

  ▸ Percutaneous drainage using CT, ultrasound, or fluoroscopic guidance is the preferred method of therapy because it provides satisfactory clinical results using local anesthesia and precludes the need for open surgical drainage

Perinephric (Perirenal) Abscess

Presenting Signs and Symptoms

Fever, leukocytosis and flank pain (at least a 2-week history of symptoms of urinary tract infection)

Frequently a history of prior antibiotic therapy with relapse on cessation

Referred pain to the thorax, groin, thigh, or hip (indicating that the disease has spread beyond the confines of the kidney)

Common Causes

PRIMARY

Forms when an intrarenal abscess breaks through the renal capsule into the perirenal space

SECONDARY

Hematogenous spread to the perirenal space from a distant focus or direct extension from an infection in an adjacent organ (e.g., ruptured appendix or diverticulitis)

Predisposing Factors

Staghorn calculus
Diabetes mellitus
Pyonephrosis
Neurogenic bladder
Immunocompromised patient

Approach to Diagnostic Imaging

▶ 1. **Computed tomography**

- ▶ Preferred study for demonstrating the low-attenuation mass (usually with an enhancing wall) as well as precisely defining the boundaries of the inflammatory process by detecting any extension into the psoas muscle and true pelvis
- ▶ Gas within the mass is virtually pathognomonic of renal abscess

 Caveat: There is *no* indication for excretory urography in the patient with a suspected renal abscess.

▶ 2. **Interventive radiology**

- ▶ Percutaneous drainage using CT, ultrasound, or fluoroscopic guidance is the preferred method of therapy because it provides satisfactory clinical results using local anesthesia and precludes the need for open surgical drainage

Pyelonephritis (Acute)

Presenting Signs and Symptoms

Rapid onset of fever and chills, flank pain, nausea and vomiting

Pyuria with white blood cell casts

Common Causes

Ascending urinary tract infection (especially *Escherichia coli*)

Obstruction is a predisposing factor (strictures, calculi, neurogenic bladder, vesicoureteral reflux)

Approach to Diagnostic Imaging

 Caveat: Uncomplicated infection requires *no* imaging; imaging studies are indicated *only* in patients who fail to respond to treatment or who are severely ill.

▶ 1. Computed tomography

▸ May demonstrate a complicating renal or perirenal abscess as a thick-walled fluid collection within the kidney that may extend to the perirenal space

---

Notes: The "pre-abscess" state of focal bacterial infection (lobar nephronia) appears as a focal wedge-shaped or rounded area of decreased density.

Uncomplicated disease appears as swollen, edematous kidneys, usually with patchy areas of decreased density or a striated parenchymal nephrogram.

▶ **2. Ultrasound**

  ▶ Also can demonstrate renal or perirenal abscess (but less sensitive than CT for detecting subtle changes in the renal parenchyma associated with uncomplicated pyelonephritis)

  ▶ Can efficiently diagnose hydronephrosis if it is unclear whether urinary tract obstruction is a predisposing factor to the development of infection

 Caveat: Excretory urography is *not* indicated to confirm the diagnosis of acute pyelonephritis or to detect complications of the disease.

Pyelonephritis (Chronic)

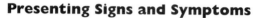

Presenting Signs and Symptoms

Progressive renal failure

History of recurrent urinary tract infections (infrequently obtained except in children with vesicoureteral reflux)

Pyuria with white blood cell casts

Common Causes

Recurrent urinary tract infections (especially when associated with obstructive uropathy)

Vesicoureteral reflux in children

Approach to Diagnostic Imaging

▶ 1. **Excretory urography**
  ▶ Demonstrates characteristic focal cortical scar overlying a blunted calyx

---

Note: Although chronic pyelonephritis is typically lobar, with normal lobes interposed between diseased ones, there may be generalized calyceal dilatation with an irregular renal margin.

▶ 2. **Ultrasound**
  ▶ Alternative approach that shows focal loss of renal parenchyma, increased echogenicity in the area of the scar, and extension of the central renal sinus echoes to the periphery of the kidney in the area of abnormality

Pyonephrosis

Presenting Sign and Symptom

Signs of infection in an obstructed kidney

Approach to Diagnostic Imaging

▶ 1. **Ultrasound**
   - ▶ Preferred screening modality for demonstrating the pathognomonic appearance of a dilated collecting system with layering of echogenic pus and debris

▶ 2. **Computed tomography**
   - ▶ May be superior to ultrasound in determining the precise site and cause of the obstruction and in defining an extrarenal abscess or fluid collection

    Caveat: Excretory urography is *not* indicated because the affected kidney functions poorly or not at all.

▶ 3. **Interventive procedure**
   - ▶ Placement of a ureteral stent or percutaneous nephrotomy catheter to relieve the obstruction (combined with antibiotic therapy) should be performed *promptly* to prevent the rapid destruction of the renal parenchyma that can result if the condition is not properly treated

Urinary Tract Infection (Infant)

Major Predisposing Factors

Obstruction of urinary tract (structural or functional)
Vesicoureteral reflux

Approach to Diagnostic Imaging

▶ 1. **Radionuclide or voiding cystography**
  - ▶ Demonstrates the presence and degree of any observed vesicoureteral reflux

---

Note: Radionuclide cystography is the most sensitive imaging technique for showing vesicoureteral reflux and delivers a substantially lower radiation dose to the gonads. It is especially valuable when multiple follow-up studies are needed to evaluate progression of disease and response to therapy.

▶ 2. **Ultrasound**
  - ▶ Preferred screening study for detecting underlying anatomic abnormalities and significant renal scarring (simple, noninvasive, no ionizing radiation)

Note: A complete investigation of the urinary tract is important after an episode of urinary tract infection in an infant because of the relatively high probability of an underlying anatomic abnormality.

▶ 3. **Excretory urography**
   ▶ Indicated if there is an abnormality shown by cystography or ultrasound to provide superior anatomic and functional information about the upper urinary tract

Note: Disadvantages in children include the ionizing radiation and need for injection of contrast material; even with good renal function, superimposition of intestinal gas and fecal material may make it difficult to evaluate the kidneys and detect focal renal scarring.

Urinary Tract Infection (Female Child)

Approach to Diagnostic Imaging

 Caveat: There is controversy as to whether female children (who constitute the overwhelming majority of those affected) should be subjected to radiographic imaging after an initial urinary tract infection (because at least 75% have no abnormality and the risk of developing reflux nephropathy in girls with normal urinary tracts at the time of their first **UTI** is very small). *But* it is generally agreed that a work-up of the urinary tract *is* indicated for repeat or relapsing infections.

▶ 1. **Radionuclide or voiding cystography**
   ▶ Demonstrates the presence and degree of any observed vesicoureteral reflux

> **Note:** Radionuclide cystography is the most sensitive imaging technique for showing vesicoureteral reflux and delivers a substantially lower radiation dose to the gonads. It is especially valuable when multiple follow-up studies are needed to evaluate progression of disease and response to therapy.

▶ 2. **Ultrasound**
   ▶ Preferred screening study for detecting underlying anatomic abnormalities and significant renal scarring (simple, noninvasive, no ionizing radiation)

▶ 3. **Excretory urography**
   ▶ Indicated if there is an abnormality shown by cystography or ultrasound to provide superior anatomic and functional information about the upper urinary tract

---

Note: Disadvantages in children include the ionizing radiation and need for injection of contrast material; even with good renal function, superimposition of intestinal gas and fecal material may make it difficult to evaluate the kidneys and detect focal renal scarring.

Urinary Tract Infection (Male Child)

Major Predisposing Factors

Obstruction of urinary tract (structural or functional)
Vesicoureteral reflux

Approach to Diagnostic Imaging

► 1. **Radionuclide or voiding cystography**
   - ► Demonstrates the presence and degree of any observed vesicoureteral reflux

> **Note:** Radionuclide cystography is the most sensitive imaging technique for showing vesicoureteral reflux and delivers a substantially lower radiation dose to the gonads. It is especially valuable when multiple follow-up studies are needed to evaluate progression of disease and response to therapy.

► 2. **Ultrasound**
   - ► Preferred screening study for detecting underlying anatomic abnormalities/significant renal scarring (simple, noninvasive, no ionizing radiation)

► 3. **Excretory urography**
   - ► Indicated if there is an abnormality shown by cystography or ultrasound to provide superior anatomic and functional information about the upper urinary tract

> **Note:** Disadvantages in children include the ionizing radiation and need for injection of contrast material; even with good renal function, superimposition of intestinal gas and fecal material may make it difficult to evaluate the kidneys and detect focal renal scarring.

Urinary Tract Infection (Older Child/Teenager)

Approach to Diagnostic Imaging

▶ I. **Ultrasound**
   ▶ A normal study indicates that there is no reflux nephropathy and that the child (by this age) is at little risk of developing intrinsic renal disease in the future

---

Note: This is the only study needed if the child has only lower urinary tract signs and symptoms.

 Caveat: There is *no* indication for excretory urography in the older child or teenager with an uncomplicated upper urinary tract infection.

Upper Urinary Tract Infection (Adult)

Presenting Signs and Symptoms

Fever
Flank pain
Pyuria

Indications for Imaging

Infection requiring hospitalization
Impaired renal function
Relapsing infection
Infection in a male

 Caveat: Uncomplicated infection in a female requires *no* imaging (and often shows no abnormalities).

Approach to Diagnostic Imaging

▶ 1. **Excretory urography**
  ▶ Provides information on structure and function of urinary tract
  ▶ Normal examination in the patient with acute urinary tract infection excludes pyonephrosis and other severe renal infections (although it does not eliminate the possibility of vesicoureteral reflux or a perinephric inflammatory process)

▶ 2. **Ultrasound**
  ▶ Preferred imaging modality for evaluating the critically ill patient with suspected upper UTI
  ▶ May demonstrate even minimal dilatation of the intrarenal collecting system, renal stones, and intrarenal masses

►3. **Computed tomography**
  ► Indicated if ultrasound or excretory urography is normal yet there is strong clinical suspicion of an infectious process involving the kidney or the perinephric space
  ► Excellent method for delineating and guiding drainage of a perinephric abscess

Renal Mass

Presenting Signs and Symptoms

Flank pain, hematuria, palpable mass, fever (suggests renal abscess)

Many are discovered incidentally in an asymptomatic patient by excretory urography, ultrasound, or CT performed for unrelated abdominal pathology

Common Causes

Cyst, neoplasm (benign or malignant), abscess

Major Imaging Goal

To separate benign renal cysts (the large majority of renal masses) from solid neoplasms

---

Note: The unequivocal imaging diagnosis of a benign cyst usually precludes the need for surgical confirmation.

Approach to Diagnostic Imaging

▶ I. **Ultrasound**
- Highly accurate for demonstrating the characteristic findings of a simple cyst:
  - Absence of internal echoes
  - Strong, sharply defined distal wall with smooth, distinct margins
  - Enhanced through-transmission of the sound beam
  - Posterior acoustic enhancement
  - Spherical or slightly ovoid shape

   Caveat: (1) Hemorrhagic or infected cysts may be indistinguishable sonographically from solid benign and malignant neoplasms and inflammatory masses, and (2) ultrasound may be inadequate in obese patients.

▶ **2. Computed tomography**
  - More sensitive than ultrasound for the detection of renal masses
  - Highly accurate for demonstrating the characteristic findings of a simple cyst as a nonenhancing mass of water attenuation with clearly defined margins, compared with a heterogeneous mass that is typical of a solid neoplasm

---

Note: Although generally considered the "gold standard" for evaluating renal mass lesions, CT is more expensive than screening ultrasound and requires intravenous contrast material. Therefore, in many centers CT is indicated only when the ultrasound examination is indeterminate or technically inadequate due to obesity or overlying gas. Because CT is more sensitive than ultrasound for detecting a renal mass, it may be used in patients with a negative ultrasound examination but a strong clinical suspicion of a renal mass. It also is appropriate to proceed directly to CT if excretory urography indicates that the renal mass is complex or likely to be solid.

 Caveat: Although renal masses are often first identified on a screening excretory urogram, this technique has a substantially lower sensitivity and specificity than ultrasound or CT for making the critical differentiation between a simple cyst and a solid, possibly malignant mass.

Renal Cyst

Presenting Signs and Symptoms

Asymptomatic (discovered incidentally during ultrasound or CT performed for unrelated abdominal pathology)

Occasionally, a palpable mass, flank discomfort or pain, or hematuria

Common Causes

Unknown

Approach to Diagnostic Imaging

Note: The imaging goal is to separate benign renal cysts (the large majority of renal masses) from malignant neoplasms, because the unequivocal imaging diagnosis of a benign cyst usually precludes the need for surgical confirmation.

Approach to Diagnostic Imaging

▶ I. **Ultrasound**
  ▶ Highly accurate for demonstrating the characteristic findings of a simple cyst
    ▶ Absence of internal echoes
    ▶ Strong, sharply defined distal wall with smooth, distinct margins
    ▶ Enhanced through-transmission of the sound beam
    ▶ Posterior acoustic enhancement
    ▶ Spherical or slightly ovoid shape

   Caveat: Hemorrhagic or infected cysts may be indistinguishable sonographically from solid benign and malignant neoplasms and inflammatory masses.

► **2. Computed tomography**

  ► Indicated if the ultrasound appearance is atypical for a simple cyst (thick wall, calcification, internal debris). Demonstrates a hemorrhagic cyst as a homogeneous mass that appears hyperdense to normal renal parenchyma on unenhanced scans and hypodense on contrast studies. Gas within a thick-walled mass strongly suggests an infected cyst.

Note: CT is indicated as the next imaging procedure if excretory urography detects a renal mass that most likely is complex or likely to be solid (rather than cystic).

Cancer of the Kidney (Hypernephroma)

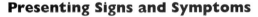

Presenting Signs and Symptoms

Hematuria
Flank pain
Palpable mass
Fever of unknown origin
Is being increasingly detected incidentally in an asymptomatic patient during ultrasound or CT performed for unrelated abdominal pathology

Approach to Diagnostic Imaging

▶ I. **Computed tomography or ultrasound**
  ▸ Screening ultrasound can demonstrate the tumor as a solid, heterogeneous, hypoechoic or mildly hyperechoic mass that may contain cystic areas representing hemorrhage or necrosis
  ▸ Contrast-enhanced CT is the most sensitive modality for detecting renal cancers

Note: Although frequently ordered as the first imaging procedure, excretory urography often misses small tumors and thus is *not* recommended as an effective screening procedure.

Staging

▶ **1. Computed tomography or magnetic resonance imaging**

> ▶ Most effective staging procedures for demonstrating the presence and extent of extrarenal spread of tumor (including invasion of the renal vein and inferior vena cava which, without distant metastases, is still a surgically curable stage of the disease)

> **Note:** Doppler ultrasound also can detect echogenic tumor thrombus within venous structures.

> ▶ MRI may prove to be accurate in determining whether the small opacities seen in the perinephric space on CT in many patients represent patent vessels or lymphadenopathy
> ▶ Chest CT should be performed for detection of pulmonary metastases prior to any potentially curative surgical procedure

▶ **2. Radionuclide bone scan**

> ▶ Should be performed to detect any skeletal metastases prior to any potentially curative surgical procedure

▶ **3. Arteriography**

> ▶ Presurgical embolization of the tumor may dramatically reduce the vascularity of the lesion, making resection easier by diminishing blood loss

Medullary Cystic Disease

Presenting Signs and Symptoms

Polyuria (with urinary sodium wasting)
Unexplained uremia
Retarded growth and evidence of bone disease
Symptoms usually begin before age 20

Common Causes

Genetic or congenital

Approach to Diagnostic Imaging

▶ 1. **Ultrasound**
  ▶ May demonstrate the multiple medullary cysts within small, smooth kidneys or merely generalized increased echogenicity of the renal parenchyma (representing diffuse atrophy)

Note: Because the cysts may be few and small, they often cannot be detected by ultrasound.

 Caveat: There is *no longer any* indication for excretory urography.

Multicystic Dysplastic Kidney

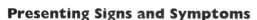

Presenting Signs and Symptoms

Palpable abdominal mass in the neonate (asymptomatic)
Usually unilateral (can be bilateral or segmental)

Common Causes

Congenital developmental defect (resulting from occlusion of the fetal ureter, usually before 8–10 weeks of gestation)

Approach to Diagnostic Imaging

▶ 1. **Ultrasound**
   ▶ Demonstrates numerous cysts of various sizes with variable amounts of intervening dysplastic renal tissue

Polycystic Kidney Disease (Adult)

Presenting Signs and Symptoms

Initially asymptomatic (may be discovered incidentally on abdominal ultrasound or CT performed for another reason)

Onset in early or middle life with symptoms related to the effects of the cysts (lumbar discomfort or pain, hematuria, infection, or colic due to nephrolithiasis)

Hypertension (50% at time of diagnosis)

Progressive renal dysfunction with uremic symptoms

Cysts may also be present in the liver (in 50%)

Aneurysms of the circle of Willis (in 15%) that may rupture to produce subarachnoid hemorrhage

Common Cause

Autosomal dominant

Approach to Diagnostic Imaging

▶ I. **Ultrasound or computed tomography**

  ▶ Demonstrates progressive replacement of the renal parenchyma by multiple noncommunicating cysts of various sizes that commonly contain internal hemorrhage

  ▶ Can detect the presence of associated cysts in the liver

 Caveat: Although excretory urography has traditionally been used to show the large irregular kidneys with compressed and elongated "spidery" renal pelvis and calyces, ultrasound and CT can make the correct diagnosis at a much earlier stage.

Polycystic Kidney Disease (Childhood)

Presenting Signs and Symptoms

In *neonates,* there is renal dysfunction with pulmonary hypoplasia (often a protuberant abdomen with huge kidneys and an enlarged liver)

In *children,* signs and symptoms of portal hypertension (due to progressive hepatic fibrosis) become more prominent and renal insufficiency is only mild or moderate

Common Cause

Autosomal recessive

Approach to Diagnostic Imaging

▶ I. **Ultrasound**
- ▶ *Prenatal* studies in late pregnancy usually can permit a presumptive diagnosis
- ▶ In young children, ultrasound shows characteristic bilaterally enlarged, echogenic kidneys with dilated renal tubules arranged in a radiating pattern (may be so dilated as to appear as individual structures)
- ▶ In older children and adolescents, ultrasound can show cysts in the kidneys and liver, as well as secondary signs associated with hepatic fibrosis and portal hypertension

---

Note: A final diagnosis may require renal and liver biopsies.

 Caveat: There is *no longer any* indication for excretory urography.

Atheroembolic Renal Disease

Presenting Signs and Symptoms

Sudden or gradual development of progressive renal failure (depending on amount of atheromatous material obstructing the renal arteries)

May have evidence of embolic disease elsewhere (cholesterol emboli visible on fundoscopic examination, neurologic deficits, toe gangrene, livedo reticularis)

Usually hypertensive

Common Causes

Spontaneous embolization of atheromatous plaques or subsequent to vascular surgery, angioplasty, or arteriography

Approach to Diagnostic Imaging

▶ 1. **Computed tomography**
   ▸ Demonstrates a resulting renal infarction as a wedge-shaped area of low attenuation within an otherwise normal kidney

---

Note: There typically is preservation of the outer 2 to 4 mm of cortex, even if the entire renal artery is occluded (because capsular branches remain patent and enhance the outer rim of the kidney).

▶ 2. **Arteriography**
   ▸ Defines vascular occlusion
   ▸ Thrombolytic therapy is less likely to be successful with embolic disease (than with acute thrombosis)

Nephrosclerosis (Malignant)

Presenting Signs and Symptoms

Severe hypertension and rapidly progressive renal failure

Common Causes

Accelerated cardiovascular disease in the course of primary hypertension (especially untreated)

May arise from secondary hypertension (due to acute glomerulonephritis, chronic renal failure, renovascular hypertension, vasculitis)

Approach to Diagnostic Imaging

 Caveat: Imaging is usually of little practical value.

▶ I. **Arteriography**
   ▸ Demonstrates increased tortuosity and more rapid tapering of intrarenal arteries and may show filling defects and loss of cortical vessels

Renal Cortical Necrosis

Presenting Signs and Symptoms

Abrupt anuria with gross hematuria and flank pain

Common Causes

In *neonates,* abruptio placenta, bacterial sepsis

In *children,* infections, extracellular volume depletion, shock, hemolytic-uremic syndrome

In *adults,* accidents of pregnancy (abruptio placenta, placenta previa, uterine hemorrhage, puerperal sepsis, amniotic fluid embolism, intrauterine death, preeclampsia), bacterial sepsis, hemolytic-uremic syndrome, hyperacute transplant rejection, burns, pancreatitis, poisoning (phosphorus, arsenic)

Approach to Diagnostic Imaging

▶ 1. **Ultrasound**
   - ▶ Initially shows enlarged kidneys; renal size progressively diminishes and may be reduced to about 50% of normal by 6 to 8 weeks

▶ 2. **Plain abdominal radiograph**
   - ▶ Demonstrates characteristic late (6 to 8 weeks) sign of calcification that is often linear and is most marked at the corticomedullary junction

Renal Infarction

Presenting Signs and Symptoms

Steady aching flank pain localized to the affected renal area

May be asymptomatic (if occlusion of a small branch of the renal artery)

Usually fever, nausea and vomiting, leukocytosis, proteinuria, and microscopic hematuria

Common Causes

Renal artery occlusion (embolic, thrombotic, arteritis, sickle cell disease)

Iatrogenic (after surgery, angioplasty, selective arteriography)

Approach to Diagnostic Imaging

▶ 1. **Computed tomography**
   ▸ Demonstrates an infarction as a wedge-shaped area of low attenuation within an otherwise normal kidney

---

Note: There typically is preservation of the outer 2 to 4 mm of cortex, even if the entire renal artery is occluded (because capsular branches remain patent and enhance the outer rim of the kidney).

▶ 2. **Arteriography**
   ▸ Defines vascular occlusion and often allows a diagnosis of vasculitis or emboli
   ▸ May be useful for thrombolytic therapy if the infarction is due to acute thrombosis

 Caveat: There is *no* indication for excretory urography because there is no renal function in the face of occlusion of the main renal artery.

Renal Vein Thrombosis

Presenting Signs and Symptoms

ACUTE (ANY AGE)

Flank pain, fever, hematuria, oliguria, edema, leukocytosis, and renal failure

SLOWLY PROGRESSIVE (ADULTS)

Gradual onset of proteinuria, deteriorating glomerular filtration rate, nephrotic syndrome

Common Causes

In *children,* diarrhea and dehydration, hypercoagulability

In *adults,* membranous glomerulonephritis, pregnancy, oral contraceptive use, trauma, extrinsic compression (lymph nodes, aortic aneurysm, tumor), invasion by renal cell carcinoma

Approach to Diagnostic Imaging

▶ I. **Ultrasound**

▸ Demonstrates an enlarged kidney in acute disease and an atrophic kidney in slowly progressive disease

---

Note: If venous collateral vessels provide adequate drainage, the kidney may be unaffected.

▸ Doppler studies may permit the direct detection of clot within the renal veins

▶ **2. Computed tomography**
  - ▸ Absence of opacification of the renal vein on contrast enhanced study

▶ **3. Magnetic resonance imaging**
  - ▸ Detection of an abnormally strong signal from the renal veins (normally a dark flow void) suggests stasis of flow
  - ▸ Slow-flowing laminar blood (paradoxical brightness) may outline a lower-signal clot within it

▶ **4. Venography**
  - ▸ The gold standard for demonstrating thrombus within the renal vein or absence of venous opacification implying obstruction

Renovascular Hypertension

Clinical Indications Suggestive of a Renovascular Cause

Onset of hypertension in a previously normotensive person older than age 50

Onset of hypertension in a person younger than age 30

Women between ages 30 and 50 who have no family history of hypertension (fibromuscular hyperplasia)

Rapid acceleration or severe hypertension

Presence of an abdominal or flank bruit

Deteriorating renal function

Poor control of blood pressure with medical therapy

Severe hypertensive retinopathy

Common Causes

Renal artery stenosis, fibromuscular dysplasia, Takayasu's aortitis

Approach to Diagnostic Imaging

Note: Many radiographic screening tests have been used in patients with suspected renovascular hypertension; there is no consensus as to which is best. Choice may reflect local institutional bias, available equipment, physician interest or expertise, and characteristics of patient population.

▶ I. **Digital subtraction angiography**
  ▸ Superior to urography for detecting renovascular hypertension. Can directly demonstrate renal artery stenosis and fibromuscular hyperplasia
  ▸ Intravenous studies less invasive than conventional arteriography but require more contrast material
  ▸ Intraarterial studies more accurate than intravenous studies and require less contrast material

▶ **2. Computed tomography angiography**
  ▸ New noninvasive technique that can demonstrate renal artery stenosis and fibromuscular dysplasia

▶ **3. Conventional arteriography**
  ▸ Gold standard for the detection of renal artery stenosis (spatial resolution of cut film is superior to digital systems)

Notes: It is infrequently used as a screening procedure because of its highly invasive nature.

Rapid-sequence (hypertensive) excretory urography was traditionally used as the screening procedure of choice to identify patients with renovascular hypertension. Positive findings included differences in renal size and rate of excretion, a delayed intense nephrogram, and extrinsic pressure on the ureter or renal pelvis from dilated collateral vessels. However, the development of alternative imaging techniques and the insensitivity of the procedure have resulted in the abandonment of the hypertensive excretory urogram.

▶ **4. Interventive radiology**
  ▸ Percutaneous renal angioplasty has become a widespread technique for the nonsurgical therapy of renal artery stenosis. The overall technical success rate is reported as 80–95%, with 10–20% of stenoses recurring (most often when there has been incomplete dilatation of the lesion). Major complications occur in about 5% of patients.

Bladder Trauma

Presenting Signs and Symptoms

Gross hematuria, lower abdominal or suprapubic pain, hypotension, pelvic fracture

Approach to Diagnostic Imaging

 1. Cystography
- Initial imaging procedure to detect extravasation of contrast material indicating intraperitoneal or extraperitoneal (more common) rupture

> **Caveat:** The urethra should *never* be catheterized if a urethral injury is suspected. Under such circumstances, the proper approach is to perform a retrograde urethrogram. Only if the urethra is shown to be normal should a cystogram be performed.

 2. Computed tomography
- In addition to demonstrating extravasation of contrast material, CT can precisely define site and extent of extraperitoneal perivesical hematoma

---

Note: CT scanning of the abdomen and pelvis is usually performed to evaluate injury to other organs after major abdominal trauma.

> **Caveat:** Bladder rupture may be missed on CT (or cystography) if the bladder is decompressed by a catheter or if it is incompletely filled. With current-generation CT scanners, the entire abdomen and pelvis may be imaged before contrast material reaches the bladder. Therefore, filling the bladder with dilute contrast through a Foley catheter or taking delayed images may be required to evaluate the bladder.

► 3. **Arteriography**
- ► Indicated in the patient with a significant pelvic hematoma who has a decreasing hematocrit and no other apparent source of blood loss
- ► Therapeutic embolization of a bleeding vessel may preclude the need for surgery

Renal Trauma (Blunt)

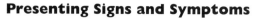

Presenting Signs and Symptoms

Hematuria

Flank pain and tenderness

Hypotension or shock

Associated injuries (skeletal fracture; signs of injury to the spleen, liver, or gastrointestinal tract)

Approach to Diagnostic Imaging

GENERAL APPROACH

1. *Unstable* patients should have immediate surgical exploration without waiting for imaging studies
2. In stable patients with *microscopic* hematuria and no suspected associated injuries or fractures, radiographic contrast studies have a very *low* likelihood of detecting significant renal injury
3. In stable patients with *gross* hematuria or microscopic hematuria and shock, the yield of radiographic contrast studies is sufficiently *high* to influence further therapy

▶ I. **Computed tomography**

  ▶ Most versatile imaging technique that can, in addition to demonstrating morphologic and functional abnormalities of the kidneys, show intraperitoneal and extraperitoneal hemorrhage, free intraperitoneal gas, and injuries to the liver, spleen, pancreas, and gastrointestinal tract

---

Note: Unsupected injuries to other organs are common and are more likely to be revealed by CT than any other imaging modality.

► **2. Excretory urography**
  ► Simple, quick, and readily available study that can be used to determine promptly whether both kidneys are present and functioning in the patient with a negative diagnostic peritoneal lavage and little likelihood of injury to other organs

► **3. Arteriography**
  ► May be indicated as a prelude to surgery in the patient with a nonfunctioning kidney that is presumed to be due to vascular occlusion

 Caveat: In 90% of cases of complete arterial occlusion, renal function is irreversibly lost after 2 hours of ischemia. Therefore, the need for immediate surgery must be balanced against the time required to complete an arteriographic examination.

  ► Embolization of a bleeding vessel may permit stabilizing of the patient before surgery

---

Note: In patients in whom iodinated contrast material is contraindicated, ultrasound may be performed to evaluate renal morphology and radionuclide scanning may be employed to assess renal perfusion and function.

Renal Trauma (Penetrating)

Presenting Signs and Symptoms

Hematuria
Flank pain and tenderness
Hypotension or shock

Approach to Diagnostic Imaging

 Caveat: In up to 6% of cases, significant occult injuries to the kidney are not suggested on clinical inspection of the wound. The absence of hematuria does *not* exclude renal injury. Studies have shown: (1) 30% of patients with penetrating flank and back trauma without hematuria had renal pedicle injuries; and (2) 15% to 42% of patients with flank or back trauma manifest only microscopic hematuria.

▶ 1. **Computed tomography**
  ▸ Contrast-enhanced scans are the imaging procedure of choice to demonstrate renal laceration and the extravasation of contrast material from the pelvocalyceal system

▶ 2. **Arteriography**
  ▸ Needed to demonstrate a bleeding vessel
  ▸ Therapeutic embolization of an actively bleeding vessel may preclude the need for surgery

Urethral Trauma

Presenting Signs and Symptoms

Inability to urinate
Blood at the urethral meatus
Elevation of the prostate on digital rectal examination
Perineal swelling or hematoma
Pelvic fracture

Approach to Diagnostic Imaging

▶ 1. Retrograde urethrography
  ▶ Imaging procedure of choice to demonstrate extravasation of contrast material through a partial or complete urethral tear

 Caveat: If urethral injury is suspected, a retrograde urethrogram should always be performed prior to transurethral bladder catheterization. If the bladder is full, suprapubic catheterization may be performed in a patient with urethral injury.

Glomerulonephritis (Acute)

Presenting Signs and Symptoms
Sudden onset of hematuria (dark urine with red cell casts), edema, hypertension, and oliguria
Elevated blood urea nitrogen and creatinine

Common Causes
Prior beta-hemolytic streptococcal infection
Other prior infection (bacterial, viral, parasitic)
Multisystem disease (systemic lupus erythematosus, vasculitis, Henoch-Schonlein purpura, Goodpasture's syndrome)

Approach to Diagnostic Imaging
▶ I. Ultrasound
  ▶ May aid in distinguishing acute disease (usually normal or slightly enlarged kidneys) from an exacerbation of chronic disease (small kidneys)

Glomerulonephritis (Chronic)

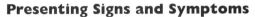

Presenting Signs and Symptoms

Insidious onset of slowly progressive impairment of renal failure associated with peripheral edema

May be discovered incidentally on urinalysis in an asymptomatic patient (proteinuria, possibly hematuria)

Common Cause

Most frequently develops weeks or months after an episode of acute glomerulonephritis

Approach to Diagnostic Imaging

▶ I. **Ultrasound**
  ▶ As with other causes of chronic renal failure, ultrasound demonstrates the nonspecific pattern of bilateral small kidneys

---

Note: Ultrasound can exclude obstructive hydronephrosis as the underlying cause of progressive renal failure.

Hydronephrosis

Presenting Signs and Symptoms

ACUTE

Colicky pain

CHRONIC

Asymptomatic or recurrent attacks of dull flank pain (resulting stasis may lead to formation of calculi and secondary infection)

Common Causes

NONOBSTRUCTIVE

Vesicoureteral reflux

Primary megacalycoces

OBSTRUCTIVE

Obstruction at the ureteropelvic junction (fibrous band, aberrant vessel, ureteral kinking, renal pelvis stone or tumor)

Distal obstruction (stone, tumor, benign prostatic hyperplasia, ureteral stricture, retroperitoneal fibrosis, bladder outlet obstruction); in pregnancy, transient involvement of right ureter

Approach to Diagnostic Imaging

▶ 1. **Ultrasound**
  - ▶ Preferred screening modality for detecting urinary tract dilatation
  - ▶ Dilatation of the renal pelvis appears as separation of the normal sinus echogenicity by anechoic urine in the collecting system

▶ 2. **Excretory urography**
  - ▶ Early signs of obstruction include a prolonged and increasingly dense nephrogram, delay in appearance of the contrast in the collecting system, and a dilated pelvicalyceal system and ureter down to the point of obstruction

▶ 3. **Computed tomography**
  - ▶ In addition to demonstrating dilatation of the ureter and collecting system, CT frequently permits identification of the cause of the obstruction

Medullary Sponge Kidney

Presenting Signs and Symptoms

Usually asymptomatic

Nephrocalcinosis may lead to such symptomatic complications as colic, hematuria, and infection (from urinary stasis)

Common Cause

Congenital dysplastic dilatation of the collecting tubules

Approach to Diagnostic Imaging

► I. **Excretory urography**
   - ► Shows characteristic striations or saccular papillary collections of contrast material (most commonly bilateral and symmetric)
   - ► Preliminary scout radiographs may show calcifications in the dilated tubules in the medullary pyramids

---

Note: Ultrasound is seldom useful because the cysts are small and located deep in the medulla (may show papillary stones as echogenic foci).

Nephrocalcinosis

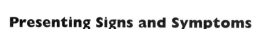

Presenting Signs and Symptoms

Asymptomatic (unless complicated by hematuria, obstruction, or infection)

Common Causes

Pathologic deposition of calcium may occur in:

Medulla
  Hyperparathyroidism
  Medullary sponge kidney
  Renal tubular acidosis
  Milk-alkali syndrome
  Hypervitaminosis D
  Hypercalcemic/hypercalciuric states

Pyramids
  Hyperuricemia
  Infection (tuberculosis)
  Sickle cell disease

Cortex
  Acute cortical necrosis
  Chronic glomerulonephritis

Approach to Diagnostic Imaging

▶ I. **Plain abdominal radiograph, ultrasound, or computed tomography**

  ▶ Although plain abdominal radiographs are the least expensive and most readily available, ultrasound and especially CT are more sensitive for detecting subtle calcification in the renal parenchyma

  ▶ Calculi appear opaque on plain radiographs, as echogenic lesions with acoustic shadowing on ultrasound, and as high-attenuation lesions on CT

Nephrolithiasis (Urinary Calculi)

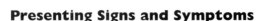

Presenting Signs and Symptoms

Asymptomatic (if not causing obstruction or passing down the ureter)

Renal colic (excruciating intermittent pain, usually originating in the flank or kidney area and radiating to the groin)

Hematuria

Chills and fever

Nausea, vomiting, and abdominal distension (clinical picture of adynamic ileus)

Common Types

Calcium oxalate or calcium phosphate (80%)

Struvite (magnesium ammonium phosphate) (13%)

Uric acid (5%)

Cystine (2%)

Approach to Diagnostic Imaging

▶ I. **Excretory urography**
   - ▶ Initial plain film of the abdomen can demonstrate the majority of urinary calculi (about 80% contain enough calcium to be radiopaque)
   - ▶ Contrast study can demonstrate lucent stones and define the precise site of obstruction and the degree of proximal ureteral dilatation

---

> **Note:** Ureteral obstruction from calculi is most likely to occur at the ureteropelvic junction or the ureterovesical junction (the narrowest points in the collecting system).

▶ 2. **Ultrasound**
   - ▶ Demonstrates both opaque and lucent stones as echodensities with acoustic shadowing, and shows the degree of ureteral dilatation proximal to an obstruction

 Caveat: Ultrasound may fail to detect small stones in the renal pelvis that do not cast acoustic shadows and thus blend in with renal sinus fat.

Tubulointerstitial Nephritis (Acute Tubular Necrosis)

Presenting Signs and Symptoms

Reversible renal failure, with or without oliguria

Symptoms vary with underlying cause (fever, rash, and arthralgias if cause is an allergic reaction to a drug)

Common Causes

Drug-induced (amphotericin, aminoglycosides, penicillins, sulfonamides, diuretics, nonsteroidal anti-inflammatory drugs, heavy metals, radiocontrast agents)

Systemic infections

Pyelonephritis

Immune disorders (transfusion reactions, transplant rejection)

Metabolic diseases (hypercalcemia, hypokalemia, hyperuricemia)

Neoplasm (lymphoma, leukemia, multiple myeloma)

Vascular (sickle cell disease, arteriolar nephrosclerosis, shock)

Crush injuries with myoglobinuria

Burns

Approach to Diagnostic Imaging

▶ I. **Ultrasound**

▶ Demonstrates nonspecific pattern of bilateral large, smooth kidneys and excludes obstruction as a cause for oliguria or anuria

 Caveat: Although excretory urography can demonstrate the prolonged bilateral nephrogram characteristic of acute tubulointerstitial nephritis, it generally is *not* required and the contrast material may aggravate the process.

Tubulointerstitial Nephritis (Chronic)

Presenting Sign and Symptom

Progressive insidious renal failure

Common Causes

Drug-induced (analgesics, especially aspirin and phenacetin)

Obstructive uropathy

Chronic pyelonephritis

Immune disorders (transplant rejection)

Metabolic diseases (nephrocalcinosis/nephrolithiasis, oxalosis, cystinosis, gout, diabetes mellitus)

Inherited multisystem disorders (polycystic disease, multicystic kidney disease, medullary sponge kidney, sickle cell disease, hereditary nephritis)

Malignancy (multiple myeloma)

Approach to Diagnostic Imaging

▶ I. Ultrasound
   ▶ Demonstrates nonspecific pattern of bilateral small, smooth kidneys

Cancer of the Urinary Bladder

Presenting Signs and Symptoms

Hematuria, pyuria, frequency, dysuria and burning

Predisposing Factors

Aniline dyes, rubber and plastics manufacturing chemicals, tobacco tars (excretory products), schistosomiasis, bladder calculi (irritative effects)

Approach to Diagnostic Imaging

▶ 1. **Excretory urography**
   ▸ May detect tumors >1.5 cm as irregular filling defects, but is less sensitive than cystoscopy

   ▼ **Caveat:** **Cystoscopic biopsy is required for histologic confirmation of the diagnosis.**

Staging

▶ 1. **Magnetic resonance imaging**
   ▸ Superior to CT for predicting the depth of bladder wall invasion (high-signal tumor disruption of the normally low-signal bladder wall on T2-weighted images)
   ▸ Equal to or better than CT for showing tumor extension into the perivesical fat (low-signal tumor vs. high-signal fat on T1-weighted images)

▶ 2. **Computed tomography**
   ▸ Alternative approach for staging if MRI not available (although not as good as MRI for differentiating superficial noninvasive tumors from those that invade the bladder muscle)
   ▸ Superior to ultrasound for defining the pelvic structures and delineating enlargement of paraaortic lymph nodes

Neurogenic Bladder

Presenting Signs and Symptoms

Partial or complete urinary retention
Incontinence
Predisposition to infection and calculus formation

Common Causes

Acute spinal cord trauma
Meningomyelocele
Diabetes mellitus
Central nervous system neoplasm (brain or spinal cord)
Cerebrovascular accident
Herniated intervertebral disc
Demyelinating process (multiple sclerosis, amyotrophic
    lateral sclerosis)
Poliomyelitis
Syphilis

Approach to Diagnostic Imaging

▶ I. **Excretory urography**
  ▶ Demonstrates marked thickening of the bladder
      wall, which has an irregular contour due to mus-
      cular trabeculation

Note: Although ultrasound also can show this appearance, it does not give any indication of the degree
of kidney function.

Bladder Outlet Obstruction

Presenting Signs and Symptoms

Partial or complete urinary retention
Progressive urinary frequency, urgency, and nocturia
(due to incomplete emptying and rapid refilling of
the bladder)
Overflow incontinence
Predisposition to infection and calculus formation

Common Causes

Benign prostatic hyperplasia
Prostatic cancer
Bladder neck obstruction (anatomic vs. functional)
Acquired bladder neck stricture (traumatic, postsurgical)
Neurogenic bladder

Approach to Diagnostic Imaging

▶ I. **Excretory urography**
  ▶ Preferred imaging technique for demonstrating the
    size of the bladder (markedly dilated or small
    and shrunken)

Note: Excretory urography can also provide valuable information concerning the functional status of
the upper urinary tracts. Characteristic findings may
suggest prostate enlargement or neurogenic bladder.
It is insensitive for detecting bladder tumors.

Cystitis

Presenting Signs and Symptoms

Dysuria, frequency, urgency
Suprapubic pain
Bloody urine

Common Causes

Infection (bacteria, tuberculosis, schistosomiasis)
Drug-induced (cyclophosphamide)
Radiation

Approach to Diagnostic Imaging

Notes: Radiographic assessment of adult *women* with lower urinary tract infection is usually of little value and rarely provides information that aids in clinical management.

Because cystitis in *men* often is associated with obstruction of the lower urinary tract, evaluation should be directed at detecting underlying prostatic or urethral pathology.

▶ 1. **Voiding cystography or excretory urography**
   ▶ Demonstrates a diffuse scalloped, irregular contour of the bladder wall and a small capacity bladder. Gas may be detected within the bladder wall in patients with emphysematous cystitis.

Urethritis (Gonococcal)

Presenting Signs and Symptoms

Dysuria
Thick, purulent urethral discharge
Primarily affects men

Approach to Diagnostic Imaging

 Caveat: Uncomplicated infections require *no* imaging (only indicated to detect complications of the disease).

▶ I. Retrograde urethrography
  ▶ Preferred technique for demonstrating the location, size, length, and number of urethral strictures as well as any periurethral communications that may be present (especially when surgery is contemplated)

Note: Retrograde urethrography is also valuable in postoperative assessment, especially in detecting residual or recurrent stenoses.

Addison's Disease

Presenting Signs and Symptoms

Weakness, fatigue, and orthostatic hypotension (early)
Increased pigmentation
Weight loss, dehydration, and hypotension (late)
Small heart size
Anorexia, nausea and vomiting, diarrhea
Decreased cold tolerance

Common Causes

Autoimmune process (idiopathic atrophy)
Granulomatous process (tuberculosis, histoplasmosis)
Neoplasm (lymphoma, metastases)
Infarction
Hemorrhage

Approach to Diagnostic Imaging

Note: Addison's disease is a clinical diagnosis that is suspected on the basis of classic signs and symptoms and confirmed by laboratory tests.

► 1. **Plain abdominal radiograph**
  ► May demonstrate adrenal calcification suggesting prior tuberculosis or histoplasmosis

► 2. **Computed tomography**
  ► May demonstrate enlargement of the adrenal glands secondary to lymphoma or metastases; idiopathic atrophy results in small adrenal glands

Adrenal Virilism (Adrenogenital Syndrome)

Presenting Signs and Symptoms

Hirsutism
Male pattern baldness
Acne
Deepening of the voice
Amenorrhea and uterine atrophy
Decreased breast size
Increased muscularity

Common Causes

Adrenal hyperplasia (infants)
Adrenal adenoma or carcinoma (adults)

Approach to Diagnostic Imaging

▶ 1. **Computed tomography**
   ▶ Procedure of choice for demonstrating the underlying adrenal neoplasm or hyperplasia

Aldosteronism (Conn's Syndrome)

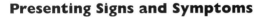

Presenting Signs and Symptoms

Hypertension

Hypokalemia

Increased serum and urine aldosterone (radioimmunoassay)

Low plasma renin activity

Common Causes

Hyperfunctioning adrenal adenoma (80%)

Adrenal hyperplasia (20%)

Approach to Diagnostic Imaging

▶ I. **Computed tomography**
  ▶ Procedure of choice for detecting the adenoma,
    which is usually small (<2 cm)

Note: Intravenous contrast is *not* needed.

Cushing's Syndrome

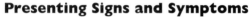

Presenting Signs and Symptoms

Truncal obesity with prominent supraclavicular and dorsal cervical fat pads ("buffalo hump")

Rounded ("moon") facies

Generalized weakness and muscle wasting

Poor wound healing and easy bruising

Hypertension

Osteoporosis

Glucose intolerance

Reduced resistance to infection

Menstrual irregularities

Common Causes

Adrenal hyperplasia (70%)
    Pituitary microadenoma (ACTH-secreting)
    Nonpituitary ACTH-secreting tumor (usually from lung malignancy)
Adrenal adenoma (20%)
Adrenal carcinoma (10%)

Approach to Diagnostic Imaging

▶ 1. **Computed tomography (abdomen)**
    ▶ Preferred screening procedure if biochemical tests suggest an adrenal tumor

---

Note: Intravenous contrast is *not* needed.

▶ 2. **Magnetic resonance imaging (pituitary)**
    ▶ Procedure of choice to detect a functioning microadenoma causing adrenal hyperplasia

▶ 3. **Plain chest radiograph**
    ▶ Preferred screening study to detect an underlying ACTH-producing lung tumor

Adrenal Metastases

Presenting Signs and Symptoms

Asymptomatic

Common Primary Tumors

Carcinomas of lung, breast, and kidney
Melanoma and lymphoma

Approach to Diagnostic Imaging

▶ 1. Computed tomography

 ▶ Procedure of choice to detect these relatively common metastatic lesions, which are often large, irregular, and inhomogeneous and invade adjacent structures

 Caveat: Small metastases tend to be homogeneous, well-defined, and indistinguishable from benign adenomas. In addition, even in patients with known primary malignancy, more than 50% of small adrenal masses are benign adrenal lesions and not metastases. Percutaneous adrenal biopsy is often needed to determine the underlying pathology.

Note: MRI may be superior to CT for analyzing small adrenal lesions because metastases (1) have a higher signal intensity than benign adenomas on T2-weighted sequences, (2) show greater enhancement than benign adenomas after gadolinium injection, and (3) do not demonstrate the presence of lipid on chemical shift imaging.

Pheochromocytoma

Presenting Signs and Symptoms

Hypertension (persistent or paroxysmal)
Tachycardia, diaphoresis, postural hypotension, tachypnea, flushing, cold and clammy skin
Severe headache and tremors
Elevated levels of catecholamines and their metabolites

Common Causes

Catecholamine-secreting tumor of chromaffin cells
  Adrenal medulla (90%)
  Extraadrenal sites (paraaortic sympathetic chain, organ of Zuckerkandl near the bifurcation of the aorta, urinary bladder)

Approach to Diagnostic Imaging

▶ I. **Computed tomography**
  ▶ Preferred screening study to detect the tumors (usually >2 cm) involving the adrenal medulla
  ▶ If no adrenal mass is found and the clinical suspicion remains high, scanning must be extended to include the remainder of the abdomen and pelvis (to search for the 10% of tumors found in an extraadrenal location)

 Caveat: Intravenous contrast material is *contraindicated.*

► 2. **Magnetic resonance imaging**
  ▶ Procedure of choice (if metaiodobenzylguanidine [MIBG] scanning not available) to search for extraadrenal pheochromocytomas (on T2-weighted images, the tumor demonstrates extremely bright signal that makes it stand out from surrounding structures)

Note: Radionuclide scans using MIBG are highly sensitive for localizing ectopic pheochromocytomas, but this agent is not widely available.

 Caveat: Arteriography is *contraindicated* in patients with suspected pheochromocytoma because of the possibility of inducing a serious and even fatal reaction.

SKELETAL

Donald Resnick

▶ SIGNS AND SYMPTOMS

Acute Monarticular Joint Pain
Polyarticular Joint Pain

▶ DISORDERS

Osteoporosis
Osteomalacia

Arthritides
Ankylosing Spondylitis
Calcium Pyrophosphate
    Deposition Disease
    (CPPD or
    Pseudogout)
Gout
Neuropathic Arthropathy
    (Charcot Joint)
Osteoarthritis
Psoriatic Arthritis
Reiter's Syndrome
Rheumatoid Arthritis

Infection
Infectious Arthritis (Septic
    Joint)
Osteomyelitis
    Direct Seeding or
        Contiguous Spread
    Hematogenous
    Vertebral

Neoplasm
Metastases (Skeletal)
Multiple Myeloma
Osteoid Osteoma
Primary Malignant
    Tumors of Bone
Soft-Tissue Tumor of
    Extremity

Other
Avascular Necrosis
Carpal Tunnel Syndrome
Congenital Hip
    Dislocation
Myasthenia Gravis
Osgood-Schlatter Disease

Trauma
Meniscal Tear (Knee)
Pathologic Fracture
Rotator Cuff Tear
Stress Fracture
Paget's Disease
Slipped Capital Femoral
    Epiphysis
Reflex Sympathetic
    Dystrophy
      (Sudeck's Atrophy)

Acute Monarticular Joint Pain

Common Causes

Gout
Calcium pyrophosphate deposition disease (CPPD)
Septic arthritis
Bursitis/tendinitis
Trauma
Hemarthrosis (bleeding diathesis)
Localized manifestation of inflammatory polyarthritis (Reiter's disease, psoriatic arthritis)

Approach to Diagnostic Imaging

▶ I. **Plain skeletal radiograph**
  ▶ Preferred study for demonstrating soft-tissue swelling and calcification, bone erosions, joint space narrowing, and any underlying fracture

Polyarticular Joint Pain

Common Causes

Rheumatoid arthritis
Ankylosing spondylitis
Reiter's syndrome
Psoriatic arthritis
Osteoarthritis
Systemic lupus erythematosus
Necrotizing vasculitis
Acute rheumatic fever
Hypertrophic osteoarthropathy
Polymyalgia rheumatica
Diffuse appearance of a usually monarticular condition
(gout, calcium pyrophosphate deposition disease,
bacterial arthritis)

Approach to Diagnostic Imaging

▶ I. **Plain skeletal radiograph**
  ▶ Preferred study for detecting soft-tissue swelling
    and calcification, bone erosions, joint space nar-
    rowing, and spur formation

Osteoporosis

Presenting Signs and Symptoms

Often asymptomatic

Dull aching pain in the bones (particularly in the lower thoracic and lumbar area)

Tendency to develop compression fractures of the vertebrae with minimal or no trauma, kyphosis of the thoracic spine, and fractures at other sites (hip, wrist) with less trauma than required in normal patients

Common Causes

PRIMARY

Postmenopausal/senile

SECONDARY (<5%)

Endocrine dysfunction

Drug-induced (e.g., steroids)

Prolonged immobilization

Chronic renal failure

Osteogenesis imperfecta

Leukemia

Approach to Diagnostic Imaging

▶ I. **Plain radiograph (spine)**

▶ May detect anterior wedging of vertebral bodies (especially in the lower thoracic and upper lumbar regions) and associated ballooning of intervertebral disc spaces that are characteristic of compression fractures

Caveat: Plain radiographs of the spine are otherwise of little value because abnormal radiolucency cannot be accurately diagnosed until at least 50–70% of bone substance has been lost.

► **2. Measurements of bone mineral content**
- ► Various methods (quantitative CT, single- and dual-photon absorptiometry, dual-energy x-ray absorptiometry) are available to assess the quantity of bone in the spine both for initial diagnosis and for following the response to therapy
- ► There is much debate concerning which imaging method is superior and even whether or not knowing the bone mineral content is clinically more helpful than mere knowledge of the age and sex of the patient (in itself fairly accurate for predicting bone-mass quantity)

Note: Most authors agree that knowing the axial bone mineral measurement does *not* help predict which patients are at risk for developing hip and vertebral body fractures.

Osteomalacia

Presenting Signs and Symptoms

Diffuse skeletal pain and bony tenderness

Bowing of long bones and loss of height of vertebral bodies (due to weight bearing on progressively weakened bones)

Common Causes

Vitamin D deficiency (lack of sunlight, dietary deficiency, or malabsorption due to chronic pancreatic insufficiency, gastrectomy, or malabsorption syndrome)

Abnormal metabolism of vitamin D (anticonvulsant therapy, chronic liver disease)

Kidney disease (chronic renal failure, renal tubular acidosis, Fanconi's syndrome)

Chronic administration of aluminum-containing antacids

Approach to Diagnostic Imaging

▶ I. Plain skeletal radiograph

   ▶ May demonstrate osteopenia (particularly in the spine, pelvis, and lower extremities) with accentuation of secondary trabeculae, thinning of the cortices, and insufficiency fractures (lucent lines running perpendicular to the long axis of the bone)

Ankylosing Spondylitis

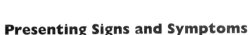

Presenting Signs and Symptoms

Recurrent back pain (often nocturnal)

Morning stiffness (usually relieved by activity)

Kyphosis (flexed posture typically eases back pain and paraspinal muscle spasm)

Chest pain and diminished chest expansion (from diffuse costovertebral involvement)

Peripheral joint pain (especially hip or shoulder)

Cauda equina syndrome

Acute iritis (anterior uveitis) in 30%

Constitutional symptoms of fever, fatigue, anorexia, weight loss, and anemia (may be severe)

Primarily affects men (3:1), especially between the ages of 20 and 40 years

Approach to Diagnostic Imaging

▶ I. **Plain skeletal radiograph**

▶ Earliest finding is erosion and sclerosis involving the sacroiliac joints in a symmetric fashion

▶ Characteristic abnormalities include squaring of vertebral bodies, syndesmophyte formation, and paraspinal ligamentous calcification that eventually produces the classic "bamboo spine"

Calcium Pyrophosphate Deposition Disease (CPPD or Pseudogout)

Presenting Signs and Symptoms

Acute attack of pain, swelling, redness, and warmth of one or more joints (especially the knee) in about 25%

Chronic progressive degenerative changes in multiple joints (at times with intermittent acute attacks)

Approach to Diagnostic Imaging

▶ I. **Plain skeletal radiograph**

- ▶ May demonstrate characteristic calcification of articular cartilage (chondrocalcinosis) in the knee, triangular fibrocartilage of the wrist, and the symphysis pubis and acetabular region

- ▶ May show structural joint changes that resemble osteoarthritis but occur in sites that typically are not involved in osteoarthritis (shoulders, wrists, and patellofemoral joints)

Gout

Presenting Signs and Symptoms

Acute gouty arthritis is an exquisitely painful mon-arthritis that typically involves the metatarsopha-langeal joint of the big toe (podagra) but also commonly attacks the instep, ankle, knee, wrist, and elbow (may be precipitated by minor trauma, over-indulgence in food or alcohol, surgery, fatigue, emotional stress, infection, or vascular occlusion)

Chronic gout is characterized by tophaceous deposits of urate crystals in joints, walls of bursae, and tendon sheaths that may lead to chronic joint symptoms, permanent erosive changes, and joint deformity

Increased serum urate concentration and hyperuricemia

Nephrolithiasis

Approach to Diagnostic Imaging

▶ I. **Plain skeletal radiograph**

  ▶ In chronic or recurrent disease, may demonstrate characteristic well-defined "rat-bite" erosions with sclerotic borders and overhanging edges (especially in the first metatarsophalangeal joints) with osteoporosis or soft-tissue tophaceous deposits (especially about the elbow, patella, and hand)

Neuropathic Arthropathy (Charcot Joint)

Presenting Signs and Symptoms

Rapidly progressive destructive process with effusion, subluxation, and instability of affected joints

Pain is often absent or less severe than would be expected from the degree of joint destruction

"Bag of bones" appearance of involved joint (due to repeated fractures and bony metaplasia that produces loose fragments of cartilage or bone)

Precise site of involvement depends on underlying disorder

Common Causes

Diabetes mellitus (foot)

Tabes dorsalis (knee and hip)

Syringomyelia (upper extremity, especially elbow and shoulder)

Spina bifida with meningomyelocele

Leprosy

Approach to Diagnostic Imaging

▶ I. **Plain skeletal radiograph**
   ▶ May demonstrate extensive destructive changes and heterotopic new bone formation

Osteoarthritis

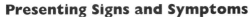

Presenting Signs and Symptoms

Insidious onset and gradual progression of pain that typically involves one or only a few joints, increases with exercise, and may become worse at night or with weather changes

Primary osteoarthritis typically involves weight-bearing (hips, knees) and frequently used joints (fingers)

Secondary osteoarthritis is due to a predisposing factor (trauma, congenital abnormality, metabolic disorder) and may be unilateral, appear at an early age, or involve joints that usually are not affected

Stiffness in the morning or after rest (usually brief)

With progressive disease, the joints may appear enlarged, motion becomes limited, flexion contractures and subluxations may develop, and tenderness and crepitus may occur

Approach to Diagnostic Imaging

▶ 1. **Plain skeletal radiograph**
   ▶ Demonstrates the typical findings of irregular or asymmetric joint space narrowing, hypertrophic bone formation (osteophytes) at the periphery of the joints, subchondral sclerosis (increased opacity), and subchondral pseudocysts (geodes)

Note: In the hands, osteoarthritis primarily involves the distal and proximal interphalangeal joints. In the wrist, the disease affects the joints at the base of the thumb. In the knee, the medial portion of the joint is more severely involved.

Psoriatic Arthritis

Presenting Signs and Symptoms

Joint abnormalities occur in about 5% of patients with skin or nail disease

Approach to Diagnostic Imaging

▶ I. **Plain skeletal radiograph**
  - ▶ Demonstrates characteristic proliferative erosions (usually affecting the distal and proximal interphalangeal joints of the fingers and toes) as well as possible resorption of terminal phalanges, bony ankylosis, or arthritis mutilans (aggressive, destructive form of the disease)
  - ▶ May be associated with spondylitis, sacroiliitis, or both (even in the absence of peripheral arthritis)

Reiter's Syndrome

Presenting Signs and Symptoms

Urethritis
Conjunctivitis
Peripheral arthritis
Mucocutaneous lesions (small painless superficial ulcers)

Approach to Diagnostic Imaging

▶ I. **Plain skeletal radiograph**
  ▸ Demonstrates asymmetric, polyarticular proliferative erosions, typically involving the lower extremities (especially the toes and the heels)
  ▸ May be sacroiliac involvement (leading to back pain), which may have a unilateral distribution

Rheumatoid Arthritis

Presenting Signs and Symptoms

Symmetric polyarthritis of peripheral joints (especially in the hand, wrist, and foot) with pain, tenderness, and swelling

Typically insidious and progressive joint involvement

Morning stiffness

Rheumatoid nodules (in 30–40% of patients)

Deformities (particularly flexion contractures and ulnar deviation of the fingers)

Carpal tunnel syndrome (due to synovitis of the wrist)

Serum rheumatoid factor

Primarily affects women (3:1) between the ages of 25 and 50 years

Approach to Diagnostic Imaging

▶ I. **Plain skeletal radiograph (hands, wrists, feet)**

▶ Demonstrates the characteristic appearance of soft-tissue swelling, periarticular demineralization, joint space narrowing, and marginal erosions that symmetrically involve the wrists and hands (primarily the metacarpophalangeal and proximal interphalangeal joints). Similar findings occur at the metatarsophalangeal joints of the feet.

> **Note:** The "rheumatoid variants" (psoriatic and Reiter's arthritis) more commonly are *asymmetric* and may involve the *distal* interphalangeal joints.

Infectious Arthritis (Septic Joint)

Presenting Signs and Symptoms

Acute joint pain associated with warmth, tenderness, swelling, and an effusion

Fever, chills, and leukocytosis

May be little systemic or local response in patients receiving anti-inflammatory drugs

Approach to Diagnostic Imaging

▶ 1. **Plain skeletal radiograph**
  ▶ Although neither sensitive nor specific, plain films may demonstrate joint effusion, joint space narrowing, and erosive changes

---

Note: The diagnosis of infectious arthritis requires a high index of suspicion (especially in patients with underlying chronic joint disease). Therefore, even the remote possibility that a joint might be septic demands aspiration of synovial fluid from an involved joint and a search of the infecting organism by Gram stain and culture (even if plain radiographs are completely normal).

▶ 2. **Radionuclide bone scan**
  ▶ Although not specific, this technique permits early diagnosis in the patient with a high likelihood of joint infection

Osteomyelitis (Direct Seeding or Contiguous Spread)

Presenting Signs and Symptoms

Pain and fever with tenderness and soft-tissue swelling

Common Causes

Trauma (open fracture, surgical reduction of closed fracture, penetrating trauma)

Bacterial contamination of orthopedic prosthesis during surgery

Diabetic or atherosclerotic arterial insufficiency of lower extremities (spread from cutaneous foot ulcer)

Sinus or dental infection (osteomyelitis of skull)

Approach to Diagnostic Imaging

▶ I. **Plain skeletal radiograph**

   ▶ May demonstrate bony destruction with the formation of lucent areas, radiopaque sequestra (foci of devitalized bone), and involucra

   ▶ An infected prosthesis may show characteristic lucent areas within the shaft of the bone adjacent to the cement about the prosthesis (may also be seen with simple loosening)

▶ **2. Computed tomography**
  ▸ Indicated to detect sequestra, which usually indicate the need for surgical removal rather than antibiotics alone (as avascular sequestra will not be effectively treated with parenteral medication)

 Caveat: Radionuclide bone scanning is of little value because the isotope accumulates in many noninfectious conditions such as fracture sites, uninfected nonunion of fractures, periosteal new bone, overlying cellulitis, neuropathic arthropathy, and aseptic loosening of prostheses.

▶ **3. Magnetic resonance imaging**
  ▸ Sensitive (but not specific) modality for detecting osteomyelitis. However, diagnostic difficulty occurs owing to the presence of bone marrow edema (neighborhood reaction) in cases of adjacent soft-tissue infection

Osteomyelitis (Hematogenous)

Presenting Signs and Symptoms

Pain and fever with tenderness and soft-tissue swelling

In *children*, most commonly involves the long bones (especially near the epiphyseal plate at the end of the shaft)

In *adults*, usually affects the vertebral bodies

Common Causes

Intravenous drug abuse

Hemodialysis

Approach to Diagnostic Imaging

▶ 1. **Radionuclide bone scan**

  ▶ Demonstrates increased activity early in the disease (evidence of bone destruction on plain skeletal radiographs usually does not appear for at least 1 week)

 Caveat: Bone scans may take months to normalize after a bone infection becomes sterile, and thus it may be impossible to distinguish a chronic infection of bone from normal healing.

▶ 2. **Magnetic resonance imaging**

  ▶ Equally sensitive or even more sensitive than bone scintigraphy for detecting hematogenous osteomyelitis, although neither technique is specific

---

Note: CT has a limited role in the early diagnosis of osteomyelitis.

Osteomyelitis (Vertebral)

Presenting Signs and Symptoms

Insidious onset and gradual progression of back pain unrelieved by heat, rest, or analgesics and worsened by movement

Fever typically is minimal or absent

Tenderness to palpation and percussion over affected bone, paravertebral muscle spasm, guarding and splinting on motion

Approach to Diagnostic Imaging

▶ 1. **Radionuclide bone scan**
   ▶ Demonstrates increased activity early in the disease (evidence of bone destruction on plain skeletal radiographs usually does not appear for at least 1 week)

    Caveat: Increased radionuclide uptake may be impossible to distinguish from that occurring with tumors and fractures.

▶ 2. **Magnetic resonance imaging**
   ▶ Although sensitive for demonstrating a focal abnormal signal intensity in the bone marrow, this modality does not accurately distinguish between infection and tumor
   ▶ Can effectively reveal the full extent of soft-tissue involvement (as can CT)

Note: Plain radiographs of the spine are not sensitive for detecting vertebral osteomyelitis. However, the findings of vertebral body destruction and rapid loss of the adjacent intervertebral disc are highly suggestive of the diagnosis of bacterial infection.

Skeletal Metastases

Presenting Signs and Symptoms

Most are asymptomatic (discovered during staging procedures)

Back pain

Common Primary Tumors

Lung

Breast

Prostate

Thyroid

Kidney

Lymphoma

Melanoma

Approach to Diagnostic Imaging

▶ I. Radionuclide bone scan

  ▶ Preferred screening technique for the detection of asymptomatic skeletal metastases, which will appear as focal areas of increased radionuclide uptake (hot spots)

  ▶ False negative may occur if there is uniform, symmetric uptake of radionuclide by diffuse metastases ("superscan"). The proper diagnosis should be suggested by decreased or no labeling of the kidneys (all radionuclide taken up by skeletal structures so that little or none remains to be excreted by the usual renal route)

► **2. Plain radiograph**
  ► If the radionuclide scan is equivocal, plain films should be obtained to confirm that a hot spot represents a metastasis rather than one of the many benign processes that can also cause increased uptake (e.g., infection, degenerative disease, trauma)
  ► Generally *not* indicated if there are multiple focal radionuclide scan abnormalities involving the axial skeleton that are virtually pathognomonic of metastases

 Caveat: *Never* order a "skeletal survey" to screen for metastases. Plain radiographs are insensitive (40–80% of cancellous bone must be destroyed before the lesion is apparent on these films).

► **3. Computed tomography or magnetic resonance imaging**
  ► Indicated to evaluate nonspecific focal abnormality on radionuclide scan or specific symptomatic areas that cannot be demonstrated or adequately characterized on plain radiographs

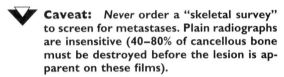 **Caveat:** Neither should ever be used as the initial screening test for suspected skeletal metastases.

Multiple Myeloma

Presenting Signs and Symptoms

Persistent unexplained skeletal pain (especially in the back or thorax)

Pathologic fractures and vertebral collapse

Renal failure

Recurrent bacterial infections (especially pneumococcal pneumonia)

Anemia with weakness and fatigue

Hypercalcemia

Excess immunoglobulins

Bence Jones protein

Approach to Diagnostic Imaging

▶ I. **Plain radiograph**

  ▶ Demonstrates either diffuse osteoporosis or multiple discrete osteolytic ("punched-out") lesions (due to replacement by expanding plasma cell tumors or elaboration of an osteoclast-stimulating factor); these lesions are often associated with pathologic fractures or vertebral collapse

  ▶ Diffuse changes may be difficult to recognize unless thinning and expansion of the cortices are appreciated

► **2. Magnetic resonance imaging**
  ► Preferred screening study to show the characteristic diffuse marrow abnormalities (low-intensity tumor replaces normal high-intensity marrow fat on T1-weighted images)
  ► In the spine, MRI can demonstrate compression of the spinal cord secondary to vertebral collapse

 Caveat: Radionuclide bone scan is *not* indicated as a screening test for multiple myeloma because the process is primarily osteolytic with little bone production (thus radionuclide scans typically are falsely normal). "Skeletal survey" is not indicated as a screening test because it is insensitive.

Osteoid Osteoma

Presenting Signs and Symptoms

Pain that classically is worse at night and relieved by
small doses of aspirin

Almost always occurs in patients younger than 30 years

Approach to Diagnostic Imaging

► 1. **Plain skeletal radiograph**
  - ► May demonstrate the characteristic appearance of
    a small radiolucent zone (nidus) surrounded by
    a large sclerotic zone (reactive bone)

► 2. **Radionuclide bone scan**
  - ► Indicated if plain film findings cannot distinguish
    osteoid osteoma from osteomyelitis. Because the
    nidus is extremely vascular, it avidly accumu-
    lates the radionuclide. This produces the typical
    "double density" sign of an area of avid radionu-
    clide uptake (nidus) surrounded by a region of
    moderately increased uptake (reactive bone), as
    opposed to a central photopenic area in osteo-
    myelitis that represents an avascular focus of pu-
    rulent material

► 3. **Computed tomography**
  - ► Indicated to define the exact location of the nidus (if
    not clearly seen on plain films) prior to surgery
    (because removal of the nidus usually results in
    complete cessation of pain)

Primary Malignant Tumors of Bone

Presenting Signs and Symptoms

Pain, soft-tissue mass

Common Types

Osteosarcoma, fibrosarcoma, chondrosarcoma, Ewing's sarcoma

Approach to Diagnostic Imaging

 1. Plain skeletal radiograph

- Preferred initial screening study (demonstration of lesion's site and appearance combined with the patient's age may permit a specific diagnosis)

Note: If a single lesion is detected that could represent a metastasis, a radionuclide bone scan (*not* a plain film skeletal survey) is essential to detect any other clinically silent lesions.

 Caveat: Although plain radiographic signs may aid in distinguishing benign from malignant lesions, none is infallible and a biopsy may be required.

2. Magnetic resonance imaging

- Best imaging modality for determining the bony and soft-tissue extent of the lesion (required prior to surgical resection)

Caveat: The ability of MRI to distinguish benignity from malignancy is controversial, and it may be impossible to determine whether high signal radiating from involved bone in some imaging sequences represents soft-tissue edema or tumor spread.

Soft-Tissue Tumor of Extremity

Presenting Signs and Symptoms

Asymptomatic and incidentally noted either by the patient or an examining physician

Variety of clinical manifestations depending on the site and type of lesion

Common Causes

Lipoma

Melanoma

Liposarcoma

Malignant fibrous histiocytoma

Approach to Diagnostic Imaging

▶ 1. **Plain radiograph**

   ▶ Although neither sensitive nor specific, this inexpensive technique is usually performed initially to demonstrate the soft-tissue lesion, its effect on the underlying bone, and any associated calcification

▶ 2. **Computed tomography or magnetic resonance imaging**

   ▶ Most accurate imaging procedures for defining the extent of a soft-tissue mass and its relationship to adjacent structures

 Caveat: **Although these techniques can sometimes suggest the nature of a soft-tissue neoplasm (especially those containing fat), a biopsy is generally required to determine the precise histologic diagnosis.**

▶ 3. **Ultrasound**
  ▶ Imaging modality of choice to determine whether a superficial soft-tissue mass thought to represent a cyst is truly fluid-filled

▶ 4. **Arteriography**
  ▶ May be indicated as a preoperative study to determine the vascular anatomy
  ▶ May be helpful in localizing an area within the mass that will most likely yield accurate biopsy data (the most malignant sites tend to have the greatest vascularity)

Meniscal Tear (Knee)

Presenting Signs and Symptoms

Pain and swelling

Click

Knee "giving way" or locking in a single position

Approach to Diagnostic Imaging

▶ 1. **Magnetic resonance imaging**
   ▶ Imaging procedure of choice for detecting partial and complete tears of the meniscus as well as associated abnormalities of the collateral ligaments and cruciates

---

Note: Arthrography of the knee is not commonly performed.

 Caveat: The need for both MRI and arthroscopy is controversial. Some studies have indicated that arthroscopy alone is sufficient and financially advisable, except perhaps in instances of recurrent knee pain following previous meniscal surgery or repair.

Pathologic Fracture

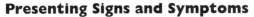

Presenting Signs and Symptoms

Evidence of a fracture following a trivial injury or without a history of trauma

Concomitant evidence of preexisting abnormality (angular deformity, painless swelling, or generalized bone pain)

Common Causes

Neoplasms (metastases; benign lesions such as simple bone cyst, enchondroma, and giant cell tumor)

Osteoporosis

Approach to Diagnostic Imaging

▶ 1. **Plain radiograph**
  ▸ Preferred initial study for demonstrating that the fracture line traverses a large area of bone destruction or that adjacent or distant bones are riddled with additional lesions

 Caveat: If the underlying lesion is small, the fracture itself may obscure the abnormal lytic or sclerotic area (especially if there is displacement at the fracture site).

▶ 2. **Computed tomography or magnetic resonance imaging**
  ▸ May be useful for detecting more subtle indications of underlying abnormal bone

Rotator Cuff Tear

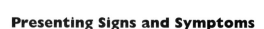

Presenting Signs and Symptoms

Pain when the arm is raised above the shoulder or adducted across the chest, but not when the arm is held down by the side

Weakness of shoulder abduction (due to underuse atrophy of the deltoid)

Approach to Diagnostic Imaging

▶ I. **Magnetic resonance imaging (shoulder)**
  ▶ Rapidly becoming the imaging procedure of choice for detecting partial and complete tears of the rotator cuff
  ▶ Noninvasive and does not require the technical expertise required for shoulder arthrography

---

Note: The imaging work-up is based on the needs of the orthopedic surgeon. If all that is needed is the detection of full-thickness tears of the rotator cuff (as opposed to partial-thickness tears), arthrography of the glenohumeral joint is generally sufficient.

Stress Fracture

Presenting Signs and Symptoms

Activity-related pain (typically associated with the repetition of a strenuous activity new or different to the affected individual) that is relieved by rest

Localized tenderness and soft-tissue swelling

Common Examples

March fracture (metatarsals in military recruits)

Lower extremity fractures in athletes, joggers, and dancers

Approach to Diagnostic Imaging

▶ 1. **Radionuclide bone scan**
   ▶ Sensitive technique for the early detection of a stress fracture

▶ 2. **Plain radiograph**
   ▶ May demonstrate a radiolucent line or a band of sclerosis associated with periosteal and endosteal thickening

 Caveat: **Plain radiographic evidence of a stress fracture may not be detectable for several weeks.**

Avascular Necrosis

Presenting Signs and Symptoms

Pain (most commonly affects the hip or knee, although the ankle, shoulder, and elbow also may be involved)

Common Causes

Trauma
Steroid therapy
Alcoholism
Pancreatitis
Collagen vascular diseases
Sickle cell disease and other hemoglobinopathies
Renal transplantation
Infiltrative diseases (e.g., Gaucher's)
Caisson's disease ("the bends")
Legg-Calvé-Perthes disease

Approach to Diagnostic Imaging

▶ **I. Plain skeletal radiograph**
  ▶ Although not sensitive, it is ideal for following the disorder from patchy sclerosis and subchondral lucency (thin line beneath the articular surface) to collapse of the articular surface, dense bony sclerosis, and joint fragmentation

▶ **2. Magnetic resonance imaging**
  ▶ Most sensitive study for detecting the earliest changes of avascular necrosis when plain radiographs and radionuclide scans are normal
  ▶ In the hip, MRI may demonstrate a characteristic low signal intensity area on some imaging sequences that virtually always involves the anterosuperior portion of the femoral head

▶ **3. Radionuclide bone scan**
  ▶ May show abnormal uptake when plain radiographs are still normal (although not as sensitive as MRI)

Carpal Tunnel Syndrome

Presenting Signs and Symptoms

Pain, paresthesias, and sensory deficits in the distribution of the median nerve

May be weakness or atrophy in the muscles controlling abduction and apposition of the thumb

Positive Tinel's sign (paresthesias after percussion of the median nerve in the volar aspect of the wrist)

Predisposing Factors

Occupations requiring repetitive hand and wrist motion

Gout

Calcium pyrophosphate deposition disease (CPPD)

Acromegaly

Myxedema

Pregnancy

Oral contraceptives

Approach to Diagnostic Imaging

▶ 1. **Plain radiograph (wrist)**
   ▶ Specific radiographic projections (including the carpal tunnel view) can permit an evaluation of the osseous structures bordering the carpal tunnel

▶ 2. **Computed tomography or magnetic resonance imaging**
   ▶ Required for assessment of the fibrous roof of the carpal tunnel and analysis of the structures coursing through the canal

Congenital Hip Dislocation

Presenting Signs and Symptoms

Inability to completely abduct the thigh to the surface of the examining table when the hip and knee are flexed (Ortolani's sign)

Hip click (audible or palpable "clunk") with abduction and external rotation of the femur (as the femoral head reenters the acetabulum)

If unilateral, shortened leg with asymmetric skin creases in the thigh

Predisposing Factors

Female infants
Breech presentation
Positive family history

Approach to Diagnostic Imaging

Note: Congenital hip dislocation is a *clinical* diagnosis.

▶ 1. **Plain radiograph (hips)**
  ▶ Although often not diagnostic in the neonatal period, plain films of the hips may be of value as a baseline study (to permit comparison with subsequent radiographic assessment as the child grows and develops)

▶ 2. **Ultrasound**
  ▶ Dynamic hip sonography (the imaging counterpart of clinical maneuvers used in physical examination) can confirm the clinical diagnosis even in the neonatal period

Myasthenia Gravis

Presenting Signs and Symptoms

Ptosis, diplopia, and muscle fatiguability after exercise
Dysarthria and dysphagia
Bulbar symptoms (alteration in voice, nasal regurgitation, choking)
Life-threatening respiratory muscle involvement (10%)
Positive edrophonium test

Common Causes

Autoimmune condition associated with thymoma in up to 30% of cases

> **Note:** A larger percentage (up to 50%) of patients with thymoma have or will develop myasthenia gravis.

Approach to Diagnostic Imaging

▶ 1. **Plain chest radiograph**
   ▶ Initial screening procedure to detect a thymoma, which appears as a smooth or lobulated soft-tissue mass that typically arises near the origin of the great vessels at the base of the heart

▶ 2. **Computed tomography**
   ▶ Most sensitive technique to detect small thymomas not evident on conventional radiographs
   ▶ Preferred method for demonstrating local invasion of tumor through thymic capsule to involve pleura, lung, pericardium, chest wall, diaphragm, and great vessels (occurs in 10–15% of patients)

 Caveat: Even CT may be unable to distinguish small thymic tumors from a normal or hyperplastic gland, especially in young patients with a large amount of residual thymic tissue.

Osgood-Schlatter Disease

Presenting Signs and Symptoms

Pain, swelling, and tenderness over the anterior tibial tubercle (at the patellar tendon insertion)

Common Cause

Trauma from excessive traction by the patellar tendon on its immature apophyseal insertion

Approach to Diagnostic Imaging

▶ I. Plain radiograph (knee)
- ▶ Demonstrates soft-tissue swelling associated with fragmentation of the anterior tibial tubercle

Paget's Disease

Presenting Signs and Symptoms

Usually asymptomatic (discovered incidentally on radiographs or routine laboratory studies)

Symptoms (typically insidious onset) may include pain, pathologic fracture of weakened bone, deformities, high-output cardiac failure, headaches, decreased hearing, and increasing skull size

Increasingly severe pain suggests fracture or sarcomatous degeneration (1% of patients)

Approach to Diagnostic Imaging

▶ 1. **Plain skeletal radiograph**
   ▶ Demonstrates cortical thickening and overall increased density of affected bones, which have an abnormal internal architecture and often show bowing or overgrowth
   ▶ Detects pathologic fractures or microfractures (tibia, femur)
   ▶ Shows areas of osteolysis in cases of sarcomatous degeneration

▶ 2. **Radionuclide bone scan**
   ▶ Most efficient method for screening multiple areas of the skeleton to search for multicentric lesions

Note: MRI and CT are the most accurate imaging modalities in the patient with suspected sarcomatous degeneration of Paget's disease.

Slipped Capital Femoral Epiphysis

Presenting Signs and Symptoms

Insidious onset of hip stiffness that improves with rest

Limp

Hip pain (radiates down the anteromedial thigh to the knee)

In advanced cases, pain present on motion of the affected hip with limited flexion, abduction, and medial rotation

May be associated with avascular necrosis and epiphyseal collapse (if compromised blood supply)

Most commonly affects overweight teenagers (usually boys)

Approach to Diagnostic Imaging

 Caveat: Early diagnosis dramatically improves the outcome because treatment becomes more difficult in advanced stages.

▶ I. **Plain radiograph (hip)**
  ▸ Demonstrates widening of the physeal line and/or displacement (posterior and inferior) of the femoral head

Reflex Sympathetic Dystrophy (Sudeck's Atrophy)

Presenting Signs and Symptoms

Pain and tenderness (usually of a hand or foot) associated with vasomotor instability, trophic skin changes, and rapid development of osteopenia

Common Causes

Local trauma
Peripheral nerve injury
Stroke

Approach to Diagnostic Imaging

▶ 1. **Plain skeletal radiograph**
   ▶ May demonstrate diffuse or patchy osteopenia of the bones of the involved extremity (especially the hands or feet)

▶ 2. **Radionuclide scan**
   ▶ Demonstrates diffuse increased uptake in the involved area (however, this finding is not specific)
   ▶ In children, foci of decreased uptake of the radionuclide may occur

NEUROLOGICAL
Burton P. Drayer

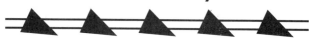

▶ SIGNS AND SYMPTOMS

Amaurosis Fugax
Carotid Bruit
  (Asymptomatic)
Dementia or Movement
  Disorder
Developmental Disorders
Headache
Seizure Disorder
  (Epilepsy)
Tinnitus
Transient Ischemic
  Attacks

Unexplained Impaired
  Consciousness
  (Stupor and Coma)
Vertigo
Visual Loss
  Unilateral Optic Nerve
    Impairment
  Optic Chiasm Lesion
  Postchiasmal Visual
    System Dysfunction

▶ DISORDERS

Infectious Processes
Brain Abscess
Central Nervous System
    Manifestations in
    AIDS
HIV Encephalopathy

Meningitis
  Acute
  Subacute/Chronic
Subdural Empyema

Neoplastic Processes
Acoustic Neurinoma
Brain Tumor
Metastases

Epidural Spinal
Intracerebral
Pineal Region Tumors

Vascular Disorders

Cerebrovascular Accident
    (Stroke)
Hemorrhage
  Intraparenchymal
    Cerebral
  Subarachnoid

Cerebral Aneurysm
Arteriovenous
    Malformation
Lacunar Infarction

Trauma

Acute Head Trauma
Epidural Hematoma
Subdural Hematoma
  Acute
  Chronic

Blow-Out Fracture of the
    Orbit
Facial Fracture
Temporal Bone Fracture
Cervical Spine Trauma

Endocrine Disorders

Acromegaly/Gigantism
Diabetes Insipidus

Galactorrhea/
    Amenorrhea
Hypopituitarism

Spinal Disorders

Herniated Nucleus
    Pulposus
Sciatica
Scoliosis
Spinal Stenosis
Failed Back Syndrome

Syringomyelia/
    Hydromyelia
Tethered Cord (Low
    Conus)
Transverse Myelitis
    (Acute)

Other Disorders

Anosmia
Bell's Palsy
Cerebrospinal Fluid Leak
Multiple Sclerosis
Normal Pressure
    Hydrocephalus
Obstructive
    Hydrocephalus

Optic Neuritis
Orbital Pseudotumor
Progressive Multifocal
    Leukoencephalopathy
Pseudotumor Cerebri
Radiation Necrosis

Amaurosis Fugax

Presenting Sign and Symptom

Ipsilateral blindness that usually resolves fully within 2–30 minutes (sudden onset and brief duration)

Common Causes

Plaques or atherosclerotic ulcers involving the carotid artery in the neck

Emboli arising from mural thrombi in a diseased heart

Approach to Diagnostic Imaging

▶ I. **Magnetic resonance imaging**

  ▶ *Imaging* of the brain is used to evaluate for infarction

  ▶ *Angiography* of the neck and head is an excellent screening study to exclude significant atherosclerotic narrowing, detect vascular occlusion, and visualize the vertebral and the anterior, middle, and posterior cerebral arteries (in addition to the carotids). If a flow gap is present (>60% stenosis), Doppler ultrasound is performed for better determination of whether the lesion falls within the surgical guidelines of 60% (Asymptomatic Carotid Artery Stenosis Trial) or 70% (North American Symptomatic Carotid Endarterectomy Trial) stenosis

▶ **2. Duplex, color-flow Doppler ultrasound**
  ▸ Most accurate noninvasive screening study that combines high-resolution, real-time imaging of the carotid arteries with hemodynamic information about blood flow velocity provided by the Doppler technique
  ▸ When used with MR angiography, may obviate the need for presurgical angiography

  Note: Other noninvasive tests (ophthalmodynamometry, oculoplethysmography) are not indicated because they cannot accurately detect carotid plaques and ulcerations.

▶ **3. Echocardiography**
  ▸ Indicated for the detection of mural thrombi in the heart if no carotid lesion has been identified that could explain the patient's symptoms

▶ **4. Intra-arterial digital subtraction angiography**
  ▸ Invasive study that provides the highest-resolution images of intraluminal vascular pathology
  ▸ Indicated prior to surgical intervention if ultrasound demonstrates a high-grade stenosis or ulcerated plaque in the carotid artery

Carotid Bruit (Asymptomatic)

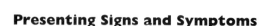

Presenting Signs and Symptoms

Asymptomatic

High-pitched sound heard over the region of the carotid artery bifurcation in the neck (must be distinguished from a venous hum, which is continuous, heard best with the patient sitting or standing, and eliminated by compression of the ipsilateral internal jugular vein)

Common Cause

Narrowing of the lumen of the extracranial carotid artery related to atherosclerotic cerebrovascular disease

Approach to Diagnostic Imaging

► 1. **Duplex, color-flow Doppler ultrasound**

  ► Most accurate noninvasive screening study that combines high-resolution, real-time imaging of the carotid arteries with hemodynamic information about blood flow velocity provided by the Doppler technique (negative predictive value exceeds 99%)

  ► Should be performed in patients with cervical bruits who are scheduled to undergo major vascular surgery elsewhere (greater than 80% carotid stenosis increases the risk of suffering a transient ischemic attack or stroke during surgery)

  ► About 20% of carotid arteries considered to be completely occluded may still have some lumen patency

---

Note: Although some advocate a battery of noninvasive tests, including ophthalmodynamometry and oculoplethysmography, these generally only add unnecessary expense.

▶ **2. Magnetic resonance imaging**
   - ▸ *Imaging* of the brain is used to evaluate for infarction
   - ▸ *Angiography* of the neck and head is an excellent screening study to exclude significant atherosclerotic narrowing; detect vascular occlusion; and visualize the vertebral, and the anterior, middle, and posterior cerebral arteries (in addition to the carotids). If a flow gap is present (greater than 60% stenosis), this Doppler ultrasound is performed for better determination of whether the lesion falls within the surgical guidelines of 60% (Asymptomatic Carotid Artery Stenosis Trial) or 70% (North American Symptomatic Carotid Endarterectomy Trial) stenosis

▶ **3. Intra-arterial digital subtraction angiography**
   - ▸ Invasive study that provides the highest-resolution images of intraluminal vascular pathology
   - ▸ Indicated prior to surgical intervention if ultrasound demonstrates a high-grade stenosis of the carotid artery

Dementia or Movement Disorder

Presenting Signs and Symptoms

Permanent or progressive decline in intellectual function
(recent memory, concentration, judgment, orientation, ability to speak or read)

Parkinsonian symptoms (including bradykinesia, rigidity, tremor)

Common Causes

Alzheimer's disease

Parkinson's disease

Multi-infarct

Metabolic/nutritional/endocrine (including Wernicke-
Korsakoff syndrome)

Brain tumor

Chronic central nervous system infection

Normal-pressure hydrocephalus

AIDS encephalopathy

Repetitive trauma (e.g., boxers)

Chronic subdural hematoma

Approach to Diagnostic Imaging

▶ 1. **Magnetic resonance imaging**
- ▶ Most sensitive examination for demonstrating large masses, hydrocephalus, and other treatable abnormalities, as well as ischemic white matter disease, small infarctions, and Wernicke-Korsakoff syndrome
- ▶ Increased iron in the corpus striatum (T2-weighted, 1.5 T studies) suggests Parkinson's disease that will not be responsive to drug therapy
- ▶ Increased signal in the globus pallidus on T1-weighted images (manganese accumulation) is seen with hepatic failure

▶ 2. **Positron emission tomography**
- ▶ Can be used as an adjunct examination in patients with suspected Alzheimer's disease because the glucose usage pattern is relatively specific

 Caveat: Because brain "atrophy" increases with age in persons with normal mental status, MRI (or CT) provides *no* reliable indication of intellectual impairment in the elderly population.

Developmental Disorders

Presenting Signs and Symptoms

Broad spectrum of neurologic deficits

Common Types

Cephaloceles
Chiari malformations
Tuberous sclerosis
Sturge-Weber syndrome
Von Hippel-Lindau disease
Cerebellar dysplasia
Posterior fossa cystic malformations (e.g., Dandy-Walker)
Neurofibromatosis
Holoprosencephaly
Migration disorders (lissencephaly, pachygyria, polymicrogyria, heterotopic gray matter, schizencephaly, abnormalities of the corpus callosum)

Approach to Diagnostic Imaging

▶ I. **Magnetic resonance imaging**
  ▶ Imaging procedure of choice to characterize and define the extent of developmental disorders of the central nervous system
  ▶ Other advantages include multiplanar imaging and the ability to image the spinal canal as well as the brain

▶ 2. **Computed tomography**
  ▶ If the patient is uncooperative and heavy sedation is contraindicated, ease of access and rapid scanning may permit performance of CT
  ▶ Useful for follow-up of shunt function

Headache

Common Causes

Increased intracranial pressure (neoplasm, abscess, hemorrhage, meningeal irritation)

Vascular disturbance (migraine, hypertension, cluster headaches)

Toxins (alcoholism, uremia, lead, systemic infection)

Trauma

Extracranial site (disorders of paranasal sinuses, eye, ear, teeth, or cervical spine)

Temporal arteritis (in elderly population)

Approach to Diagnostic Imaging

▶ **I. Magnetic resonance imaging**

▶ Most sensitive technique for detecting cerebral lesions responsible for headache (especially in patients who have coexistent abnormal neurologic signs)

▶ Imaging evaluation is usually unnecessary in patients with no neurologic abnormalities and who have either continuous headaches of long duration (many months or years) or intermittent recurrent headaches

 Caveat: Patients with severe *acute* headaches should be imaged with noncontrast head CT because of the suspicion of subarachnoid hemorrhage, acute hydrocephalus, or an enlarging intracranial mass.

Note: There is *no* indication for conventional skull radiographs. If disease of the paranasal sinuses is suspected, a limited coronal CT study can be performed.

Seizure Disorder (Epilepsy)

Presenting Signs and Symptoms

Sudden brief attacks of altered consciousness, motor activity, sensory phenomena, or inappropriate behavior

Common Causes

Congenital or developmental brain defects (usually onset of seizures at an early age)

Idiopathic (typically begins between ages 2 and 18)

Acute infection (febrile convulsion in child)

Trauma

Brain tumor

Metabolic disturbance (hypoglycemia, uremia, hepatic failure, electrolyte abnormality)

Toxic agent (lead, alcohol, cocaine)

Cerebral infarction or hemorrhage

Mesial temporal sclerosis

Approach to Diagnostic Imaging

► I. **Magnetic resonance imaging**
  ► Most sensitive screening technique for detecting underlying cerebral abnormality (indicated in all adults with an unexplained first seizure)
  ► Follow-up MRI (at 3–6 months) is often of value if the initial examination failed to detect a source of the seizure disorder

---

Note: Examination consists of a routine brain study plus high-resolution, thin-section (2–3 mm) coronal T2-weighted images.

►**2. Positron emission tomography**
  ► Using F-18 deoxyglucose, this modality improves localization of the seizure focus, particularly in the patient with complex partial (temporal lobe), medically intractable seizures who has had a normal MRI scan

►**3. Computed tomography**
  ► Noncontrast scan is recommended as the initial study if the patient is in the immediate postictal state, or if residual neurologic deficit is present at the time of imaging

---

Note: In pediatric patients, contrast enhancement is generally not required because congenital anomalies, rather than tumor, are the most common structural cause of seizures.

Tinnitus

Presenting Signs and Symptoms

Perception of sound in the absence of an acoustic stimulus (ringing, buzzing, roaring, whistling, hissing) that may be intermittent, continuous, or pulsatile

Often an associated hearing loss

Common Causes

Virtually any ear disorder (obstruction, infection, cholesteatoma, neoplasm, eustachian tube obstruction, otosclerosis)

Cerebellopontine angle tumor

Drugs (salicylates, quinine, alcohol, certain antibiotics and diuretics)

Cardiovascular disease (hypertension, arteriosclerosis, aneurysms)

Trauma

Approach to Diagnostic Imaging

▶ 1. **Computed tomography (of temporal bone)**
  ▶ Preferred study for showing morphologic abnormality of ear bones

> **Note:** Thin (1.5 mm) sections in axial and coronal planes are required.

► **2. Magnetic resonance imaging**
  ► If CT fails to detect a cause of symptoms, high-resolution, thin-section MRI is the preferred study for demonstrating small tumors (e.g., neurinoma) of the intracanalicular portion of the 8th cranial nerve as well as vascular abnormalities in the region of the cerebellopontine angle
  ► Contrast infusion is often used, although the need for it may be obviated if thin-section (2–3 mm), axial, and coronal T1-weighted and coronal T2-weighted fast spin echo images are obtained

Transient Ischemic Attacks

Presenting Sign and Symptom

Focal neurologic deficit that resolves fully within 24 hours (sudden onset and brief duration)

Common Causes

Plaques or atherosclerotic ulcers involving the carotid or vertebral arteries in the neck

Emboli arising from mural thrombi in a diseased heart

Approach to Diagnostic Imaging

Note: The following results of clinical trials indicate the need to accurately detect carotid artery stenosis: (1) North American Symptomatic Carotid Endarterectomy Trial (NASCET) study confirms the value of carotid endarterectomy for stenosis (>70%) to prevent stroke and improve quality of life; (2) Asymptomatic Carotid Artery Stenosis Trial (ACAS) study suggests surgery to prevent stroke for carotid stenosis (>60%).

▶ I. **Duplex, color-flow Doppler ultrasound**
   ▸ Accurate noninvasive screening study that combines high-resolution, real-time imaging of the carotid arteries with hemodynamic information about blood flow velocity provided by the Doppler technique
   ▸ When used with magnetic resonance angiography, may obviate the need for presurgical arteriography

Note: Other noninvasive tests (ophthalmodynamometry, oculoplethysmography) are not indicated because they cannot accurately detect carotid plaques and ulcerations.

▶ **2. Magnetic resonance angiography**
- ▸ Accurate noninvasive screening study for detecting not only disease of the carotid bifurcation, but also narrowing of the vertebral arteries. Reconstitution sign (flow gap) confirms greater than 60% stenosis (i.e., surgical disease)
- ▸ If surgery is contemplated, brain MR imaging and angiography can complete the diagnostic workup and preclude the need for catheter arteriography

▶ **3. Echocardiography**
- ▸ Indicated for the detection of mural thrombi in the heart if no carotid lesion has been identified that could explain the patient's symptoms

▶ **4. Intra-arterial digital subtraction angiography**
- ▸ Invasive study that provides the highest-resolution images of intraluminal vascular pathology
- ▸ Indicated prior to surgical intervention if ultrasound demonstrates a high-grade stenosis or ulcerated plaque in the carotid artery

Unexplained Impaired Consciousness (Stupor and Coma)

Presenting Signs and Symptoms

Vigorous stimuli required to elicit a response (stupor)
Unarousable unresponsiveness (coma)

Common Causes

Trauma (diffuse cerebral edema; epidural, subdural, intraparenchymal, or subarachnoid hemorrhage)
Anoxia or ischemia (stroke, syncope)
Epilepsy (postictal state)
Exogenous toxins (alcohol, hypnotics, narcotics)
Endogenous toxins (uremia, hepatic coma, diabetic acidosis, hypoglycemia, hyponatremia)
Brain tumor, infarction, abscess, or meningitis

Approach to Diagnostic Imaging

▶ I. Computed tomography
  ▶ Can rapidly determine whether there is extra-axial hemorrhage, mass lesion, or herniation requiring emergency surgical decompression

 Caveat: Because patients with disordered consciousness due to high intracranial pressure can deteriorate rapidly, do not delay therapy if CT cannot be obtained promptly.

► **2. Magnetic resonance imaging**
  ► Procedure of choice in *subacute* phase for better visualization of the temporal lobes (e.g., herpes encephalitis), brain stem (e.g., central pontine myelinolysis), white matter (e.g., gliomatosis cerebri), and superior calyculi and mammillary bodies (Wernicke's)

Note: Plain skull radiographs are of no value and should *not* be obtained.

Vertigo

Presenting Signs and Symptoms

Impression of movement in space or objects, loss of equilibrium, nausea and vomiting, nystagmus

Common Causes

Labyrinthine or middle ear infection or tumor
Head trauma
Toxic agent (alcohol, opiates, streptomycin)
Meniere's disease
Cerebellopontine angle tumor (neurinoma, meningioma, metastasis, epidermoid)
Transient vertebrobasilar ischemic attacks
Motion sickness
Multiple sclerosis (focal brain stem lesion)

Approach to Diagnostic Imaging

▶ 1. **Magnetic resonance imaging**
   ▶ Preferred study for detecting abnormalities of the posterior fossa and cerebellopontine angle (using high-resolution, thin-section MRI)
   ▶ Contrast enhancement is helpful for detecting a small acoustic neurinoma

> **Note:** If paramagnetic contrast material is not used, an additional thin-section, coronal T2-weighted fast spin echo sequence should be obtained.

▶ 2. **Computed tomography**
   ▶ Indicated if middle ear pathology is suspected

> **Note:** Thin-section (1.5 mm) scanning in the axial and coronal planes using a bone-highlighting algorithm is required.

Visual Loss: Unilateral Optic Nerve Impairment

Presenting Signs and Symptoms

Purely monocular visual loss

Normal ocular examination (or only optic atrophy) of both the symptomatic and asymptomatic eye

Common Causes

Optic neuritis

Ischemic optic neuropathy

Compressive-infiltrative optic neuropathies (optic nerve glioma, lymphoma, leukemia, sarcoidosis)

Extrinsic compression by orbital mass (meningioma, metastasis)

Orbital pseudotumor

Thyroid exophthalmopathy

Approach to Diagnostic Imaging

► 1. **Computed tomography**
   - ► Axial 3-mm sections provide clear distinction of the optic nerves, extraocular muscles, and globe. Because CT is superb for detecting the presence of calcification (very useful in the differential diagnosis of orbital masses) and orbital fat provides excellent contrast, some recommend this modality as the initial and often the definitive imaging study for orbital pathology.

► 2. **Magnetic resonance imaging**
   - ► Advantage of multiplanar imaging

Note: Contrast enhancement and fat suppression generally are required for the detection of orbital masses.

Visual Loss: Optic Chiasm Lesion

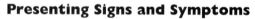

Presenting Signs and Symptoms

Bitemporal visual field defects (although deficit may be substantially greater in one eye than in the other)

Common Causes

Pituitary tumor

Parasellar mass (meningioma, craniopharyngioma, aneurysm)

Approach to Diagnostic Imaging

▶ 1. **Magnetic resonance imaging**

    ▸ Preferred study for detecting a lesion compressing the optic chiasm because of its ability to image the sella and parasellar regions in the axial, coronal, and sagittal planes

    ▸ Can clearly demonstrate the entire course of the optic nerves, optic chiasm, and optic radiations as well as the cavernous sinuses and carotid arteries

Visual Loss: Postchiasmal Visual System Dysfunction

Presenting Signs and Symptoms

Bilateral homonymous hemianopia (visual field defects on same side of the vertical median for each eye)

Normal visual acuity, pupillary reflexes, and ophthalmoscopy

Common Causes

Tumor (primary or metastatic)

Abscess

Infarction

Arteriovenous malformation

Hematoma

Approach to Diagnostic Imaging

▶ I. **Magnetic resonance imaging**
   ▶ Preferred study for evaluating the optic tracts, optic radiations, and visual cortex

---

Note: T1-, intermediate-, and T2-weighted axial images are usually sufficient.

Brain Abscess

Presenting Signs and Symptoms

Headache
Nausea and vomiting
Papilledema
Lethargy
Seizures
Focal neurologic deficits
Fever, chills, and leukocytosis

Common Causes

Direct extension of cranial infection (osteomyelitis, mastoiditis, sinusitis, subdural empyema)
Penetrating trauma
Hematogenous spread (bacterial endocarditis, IV drug abuse, bronchiectasis, congenital heart disease with right-to-left shunt)

Approach to Diagnostic Imaging

▶ 1. **Magnetic resonance imaging**
  ▶ Most sensitive study for detecting the typically ring-enhancing mass lesion and associated edema and mass effect
  ▶ Superior to CT for detecting multiple brain abscesses
▶ 2. **Computed tomography**
  ▶ Contrast-enhanced study can identify the high-attenuation capsule surrounding the hypodense necrotic center (if MRI is not available)

Central Nervous System Manifestations in AIDS

Presenting Signs and Symptoms

Spectrum of neurologic deficits depending on region and extent of involvement

Common Causes

HIV encephalitis
Cytomegalovirus
Toxoplasmosis
Cryptococcosis
Lymphoma
Progressive multifocal leukoencephalopathy (PML)

Approach to Diagnostic Imaging

► I. **Magnetic resonance imaging**
  ► Most sensitive screening study in symptomatic patients for demonstrating single or multiple lesions of abnormal signal intensity or diffuse changes in the deep white matter
  ► If nonenhanced MRI is positive, contrast enhancement is helpful in differentiating abscess and lymphoma (enhance) from HIV encephalitis and PML (no enhancement)

HIV Encephalopathy

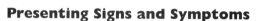

Presenting Signs and Symptoms

Progressive encephalopathy, somnolence, slow speech, word-finding difficulty, flat affect, and diminished attention in an HIV-positive patient

Approach to Diagnostic Imaging

▶ I. **Magnetic resonance imaging**

▶ In addition to showing central atrophy out of proportion to the patient's age, this modality is the most sensitive for demonstrating high-signal lesions (on T2-weighted images) that are focally or diffusely distributed throughout the deep white matter

> **Note:** Although there is poor correlation between the extent of atrophy and the severity of the dementia in AIDS, symptomatic HIV-positive patients are more than three times as likely to have abnormal MRI examinations. Routine MRI screening of neurologically asymptomatic HIV-positive patients is *not* cost-effective. When an abnormality is found on nonenhanced MRI, the use of paramagnetic contrast material assists in distinguishing HIV encephalitis and progressive multifocal leukoencephalopathy (which do *not* enhance) from abscess and primary central nervous system lymphoma (which *do* enhance).

Acute Bacterial Meningitis

Presenting Signs and Symptoms

Prodromal respiratory illness or sore throat, headache, stiffneck, fever, vomiting, seizures, impaired consciousness

Common Organisms

Meningococcus, *Haemophilus influenzae* (type b), pneumococcus, Gram-negative organisms

Common Causes

Extension from nearby infected structures (sinusitis, epidural abscess)

Communication of cerebrospinal fluid with exterior (penetrating trauma, myelomeningocele, spinal dermal sinus, neurosurgical procedures)

Approach to Diagnostic Imaging

► **1. Computed tomography (head)**
  - ► Contrast scans may demonstrate characteristic enhancement of the subarachnoid spaces in addition to small ventricles and effacement of the sulci secondary to cerebral edema
  - ► May demonstrate the underlying cause for the development of meningitis (brain abscess, sinus or mastoid infection, congenital anomaly)
  - ► Most important role of imaging is to exclude a mass (abscess) prior to performing a lumbar puncture (the primary diagnostic test)

Note: MRI may be normal in patients with meningitis if contrast material is not used.

 Caveat: Because acute bacterial meningitis (especially meningococcal) can be rapidly lethal, do *not* delay use of antibiotics pending results of diagnostic tests.

Subacute/Chronic Meningitis

Presenting Signs and Symptoms

Similar to acute bacterial meningitis (but developing over weeks rather than days)

Common Causes

Chronic infection (fungal, tuberculosis, syphilis, amebic)
Immunosuppressive therapy
AIDS
Neoplasm (leukemia, lymphoma, melanoma, carcinomas, gliomas)
Sarcoidosis
Lyme disease

Approach to Diagnostic Imaging

▶ 1. **Magnetic resonance imaging**
  - ▶ Contrast scans are required to demonstrate characteristic enhancement of the subarachnoid spaces as well as an underlying neoplasm
  - ▶ Can demonstrate associated brain edema, abscess, or neoplasm as well as inflammation of the paranasal sinuses or mastoids

▶ 2. **Plain chest radiograph**
  - ▶ Indicated to search for evidence of underlying tuberculosis or sarcoidosis

Subdural Empyema

Presenting Signs and Symptoms

Headache
Lethargy, vomiting, and fever
Focal neurologic deficits
Seizures
Often rapid clinical deterioration (an emergency condition)

Common Causes

Extension from nearby infected structure (sinusitis, ear infection, osteomyelitis, brain abscess)
Penetrating trauma
Surgical drainage of a subdural hematoma
Bacteremia (especially from pulmonary infection)

Approach to Diagnostic Imaging

▶ I. **Computed tomography or magnetic resonance imaging**
   ▶ Demonstrates characteristic crescentic or lentiform extra-axial fluid collection that is of low attenuation on CT and mildly hyperintense to cerebrospinal fluid on T2-weighted MRI
   ▶ Contrast studies show the intensely enhancing surrounding membrane

Note: Subdural empyema is far easier to visualize using MRI (because it can be extremely difficult on CT to detect the extracerebral collection adjacent to the skull unless wider windowing is used).

Acoustic Neurinoma

Presenting Signs and Symptoms

Hearing loss (sensorineural)
Tinnitus
Dizziness and unsteadiness

Approach to Diagnostic Imaging

▶ 1. **Magnetic resonance imaging**
  ▶ Preferred study for detecting abnormalities of the cerebellopontine angle and posterior fossa
  ▶ Small intracanalicular tumors may be identified because of their intense contrast enhancement

---

Note: A thin-section, multiplanar, high-resolution study is required.

▶ 2. **Computed tomography**
  ▶ Indicated if there is conductive hearing loss to evaluate bony abnormality in the petrous portion of the temporal bone

---

Note: Thin sections with bone windows are required.

Brain Tumor

Presenting Signs and Symptoms

Slowly progressive focal neurologic deficits (depending on the site of the lesion)

Nonfocal symptoms due to increased intracranial pressure

Seizures

Mental symptoms (drowsiness, lethargy, personality changes, impaired mental faculties, psychotic episodes)

Signs of herniation

Approach to Diagnostic Imaging

▶ I. **Magnetic resonance imaging**

- ▶ Preferred screening technique for detecting and characterizing intracranial masses (may not require contrast infusion)

- ▶ Surgical planning or tumor biopsy can be performed using an MRI-compatible stereotaxic frame

Note: CT is only indicated to demonstrate bone erosion (especially at the skull base) and intramass calcification (although gradient-recalled echo sequences increase the sensitivity of MRI to calcification), and for CT-guided biopsy.

Epidural Spinal Metastases

Presenting Signs and Symptoms

Back pain

Progressive weakness and sensory symptoms (numbness and paresthesias)

Bowel and bladder dysfunction

Corticospinal tract signs

Common Primary Neoplasms

Lung, breast, prostate, melanoma, lymphoma, kidney, gastrointestinal tract

Approach to Diagnostic Imaging

▶ **I. Plain spinal radiograph**

- ▸ Demonstrates single or multiple, lytic or blastic lesions or compression fractures in 60–85% of patients with epidural metastases
- ▸ Ineffective for detecting early metastases because about 50% of cancellous bone in the region must be destroyed before lytic lesions show on plain radiographs

▶ **2. Magnetic resonance imaging**

- ▸ Most sensitive technique that can simultaneously demonstrate the bone marrow abnormalities of vertebral metastases (hypointense on T1-weighted images and hyperintense on T2-weighted scans) and epidural extension effacing and displacing the spinal cord and nerve roots

Note: Differentiation of benign from malignant causes of vertebral body fracture can be accomplished by MRI. Factors consistent with malignancy include complete (or nearly so) tumor replacement of marrow in vertebral bodies and posterior elements, multilevel involvement, and paravertebral masses.

 Caveat: Contrast enhancement may obscure evidence of destructive changes in the vertebral bodies.

Intracerebral Metastases

Presenting Signs and Symptoms

Headache
Focal neurologic deficits
Drowsiness
Papilledema
Seizures

Common Primary Neoplasms

Lung
Breast
Melanoma
Gastrointestinal tract
Kidney

Approach to Diagnostic Imaging

▶ I. **Magnetic resonance imaging**
  - ▶ Nonenhanced MRI is extremely sensitive for detecting brain metastases (predominantly located at the grey-white junction)
  - ▶ Contrast enhancement makes this modality even more sensitive for the detection of brain metastases
  - ▶ Associated vasogenic edema that is seen on T2-weighted images consists of pure edema with no tumor extension

---

Note: Enhanced CT is limited by artifacts in the temporal lobes and posterior fossa.

Pineal Region Tumors

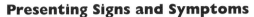

Presenting Signs and Symptoms

Precocious puberty (especially in boys)

Paralysis of upward gaze (Parinaud's syndrome relating to compression of tectal plate)

Noncommunicating hydrocephalus (due to obstruction at the aqueduct of Sylvius)

Papilledema and other signs of increased intracranial pressure

Common Causes

Germinoma

Teratoma

Glioma

Approach to Diagnostic Imaging

▶ 1. **Magnetic resonance imaging**

  ▶ Most sensitive study for detecting a neoplasm in the pineal region, but is rarely specific enough to provide a histologic diagnosis (except for the heterogenous appearance of intratumoral fat and calcium in a teratoma)

  ▶ Combination of axial and sagittal images permits visualization of even small tumors. Obstruction of the aqueduct may obliterate the normal pulsatile signal void

  ▶ A benign pineal cyst may measure up to 25 mm and have a signal intensity not precisely the same as that of cerebrospinal fluid. The benign nature of the lesion is confirmed by the absence of obstructive hydrocephalus and the unchanging size on serial examinations

 Caveat: Enhancement may occur normally in the pineal region. This appearance should *not* be mistaken for tumor enhancement.

Cerebrovascular Accident (Stroke)

Presenting Signs and Symptoms

Abrupt, dramatic onset of focal neurologic deficit that does not resolve within 24 hours

Possible headache or seizure

Common Causes

Infarction (secondary to an embolism from the heart or extracranial circulation or to hemorrhage)

Narrowing of intracranial or extracranial artery (atherosclerosis, thrombus, dissection, vasculitis)

Thrombus of the cerebral venous system

Rupture of an aneurysm or arteriovenous malformation (causing subarachnoid hemorrhage or intracerebral hematoma)

Decreased perfusion pressure or increased blood viscosity with inadequate blood flow reaching the brain

Approach to Diagnostic Imaging

▶ I. Computed tomography

  ✓ ▶ Noncontrast study is the preferred initial procedure for assessing a suspected acute stroke because it can rule out hemorrhage (subarachnoid or intracerebral), define patterns of ischemic injury, show areas of abnormal vascular calcification (e.g., giant aneurysm), and exclude a mass lesion

---

Note: The above information is critical for the clinician faced with determining the need for lumbar puncture, vascular surgery, anticoagulation, or other therapies.

▶ **2. Magnetic resonance imaging**
    ▶ The combination of nonenhanced MR imaging and angiography is more sensitive than CT for detecting infarction and ischemic edema (especially involving the brainstem), clearly delineating an occluded or stenotic artery or vein, and distinguishing hemorrhagic from ischemic infarction

 Caveat: Arteriography is indicated *only* if noninvasive studies suggest an underlying aneurysm or AVM *and* a surgical or interventive radiologic procedure is seriously considered.

Intraparenchymal Cerebral Hemorrhage

Presenting Signs and Symptoms

Abrupt onset of headache followed by steadily increasing
  neurologic deficits
Loss of consciousness
Nausea, vomiting, and delirium
Focal or generalized seizures
Signs of transtentorial herniation

Common Causes

Trauma
Hypertensive hematoma (common locations: putamen-
  external capsule, caudate, thalamus, pons, cerebel-
  lum, cerebral hemisphere)
Congenital aneurysm or arteriovenous malformation
Amyloid angiopathy (causes polar hemorrhage)
Mycotic aneurysm
Blood dyscrasia (bleeding diathesis)
Collagen disease
Hemorrhagic infarction (gyral hemorrhage)

Approach to Diagnostic Imaging

▶ I. **Computed tomography**
- ▸ Preferred imaging technique for detecting a focal region of increased attenuation within the brain parenchyma in *acute* trauma or suspected aneurysm rupture (because of superior detection of subarachnoid hemorrhage and patient comfort)

 Caveat: Although it is unusual, CT may at times fail to detect subarachnoid blood found at lumbar puncture.

▶ 2. **Magnetic resonance imaging**
- ▸ Preferred study for detecting *subacute* and *chronic* stages of intraparenchymal hemorrhage
- ▸ Hemosiderin- or ferritin-laden macrophages that develop due to prior bleeding appear as hypointense foci on T2-weighted images and persist throughout the patient's life

Subarachnoid Hemorrhage

Presenting Signs and Symptoms

Sudden onset of excruciating headache

Rapid loss of consciousness

Vomiting

Severe neck stiffness (usually not present initially but occurring within 24 hours)

Progressive palsies (reflecting pressure effects on the 3rd, 4th, 5th, and 6th cranial nerves)

Common Causes

Trauma

Rupture of congenital intracranial aneurysm

Arteriovenous malformation (AVM)

Mycotic aneurysm (in patients with infective endocarditis or systemic infection or who are immunocompromised)

Blood dyscrasia (bleeding diathesis)

Approach to Diagnostic Imaging

▶ I. **Computed tomography**
  - ▶ Preferred study for demonstrating acute subarachnoid hemorrhage
  - ▶ Initial noncontrast scan to detect the presence of high-attenuation blood in the subarachnoid space
  - ▶ Subsequent contrast-enhanced CT or MRI/MRA may detect the underlying aneurysm or vascular malformation

 Caveat: Lumbar puncture to demonstrate blood in the subarachnoid space is indicated *only* if CT fails to make the diagnosis *and* shows no evidence of a mass or obstructive hydrocephalus (lest herniation occur).

▶2. Arteriography
- ▸ Indicated to localize and characterize the anatomy of an aneurysm or AVM
- ▸ If there is an aneurysm, must also evaluate for vasospasm

---

> **Note:** Must selectively catheterize (or, less optimally, reflux contrast material into) both carotid and both vertebral arteries.

▶3. Magnetic resonance imaging
- ▸ Superior to CT for demonstrating *subacute* and *chronic* subarachnoid hemorrhage
- ▸ Relatively insensitive to subarachnoid hemorrhage in the *acute* stage
- ▸ Role of MRA in aneurysm detection is emerging, although the gold standard remains selective catheter arteriography

Cerebral Aneurysm

Presenting Signs and Symptoms

Asymptomatic

Signs of intraparenchymal or subarachnoid hemorrhage (if rupture)

Compression of cranial nerves or brain parenchyma (if large)

Common Causes

Congenital (berry)

Atherosclerotic

Mycotic

Traumatic

Approach to Diagnostic Imaging

▶ 1. **Computed tomography**
   ▶ To detect subarachnoid hemorrhage and intracerebral hematoma

▶ 2. **Arteriography**
   ▶ If the clinical suspicion of a cerebral aneurysm has been suggested by CT or MRI evidence of intraparenchymal or subarachnoid hemorrhage, arteriography can identify the presence of any and all aneurysms, delineate the relationship of a given aneurysm to the parent vessel and adjacent penetrating branches, define the potential for collateral circulation to the brain, and assess for vasospasm

►3. **Computed tomography or magnetic resonance imaging**
  - ► Can demonstrate a patent suprasellar aneurysm as an intensely enhancing mass (CT) or as a high-velocity flow void with signal heterogeneity due to turbulence (MRI)

►4. **Magnetic resonance angiography**
  - ► Demonstrates the parent artery and depicts the size and orientation of the neck and dome of the aneurysm
  - ► Future technical refinements will permit detection of progressively smaller aneurysms
  - ► Useful screening study in asymptomatic patients, as well as in those with a family history of aneurysms or a familial disorder associated with cerebral aneurysms

Arteriovenous Malformation (AVM)

Presenting Signs and Symptoms

Asymptomatic

Sudden headache and neurologic deficits (secondary to intraparenchymal or subarachnoid hemorrhage)

Focal seizures (incited by the lesion)

Progressive focal neurologic sensory-motor deficit (due to enlarging AVM acting as a mass or progressive ischemic lesion)

May have arterial bruit detectable on the overlying cranial vault

Common Cause

Congenital tangle of dilated blood vessels with direct flow from arterial afferents into venous efferents

Approach to Diagnostic Imaging

▶ 1. **Magnetic resonance imaging**

  ▸ Demonstrates AVMs as tangled flow voids with prominent feeding and draining vessels

  ▸ Superior to CT for demonstrating *subacute* and *chronic* hemorrhage and secondary changes (mass effect, edema), as well as ischemic changes in the adjacent brain

  ▸ Optimal for detecting low-flow and angiographically occult vascular malformations (cavernous angioma, telangiectasia, venous angioma)

▶ 2. **Arteriography**

  ▸ Required to precisely demonstrate the anatomic blood supply and drainage prior to any surgical or neurointerventional procedure

  ▸ Can distinguish among pial, dural, and mixed types of AVMs

Lacunar Infarction

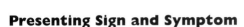

Presenting Sign and Symptom

Focal neurologic deficit that can be pinpointed to a locus less than 15 mm in diameter

Common Causes

Embolic, atherosclerotic, or thrombotic lesions in long single penetrating end-arterioles supplying the deep cerebral white matter, thalamus, basal ganglia-capsular region, and pons

Hypertension is common

Approach to Diagnostic Imaging

▶ I. **Magnetic resonance imaging**

  ▶ *Only* modality that can consistently demonstrate the well-delineated round or slit-like lesions that are hypointense to brain on T1-weighted images and hyperintense to brain on intermediate and T2-weighted images

---

Note: Because of their small size, most true lacunar infarctions cannot be seen on CT scans.

  ▶ Magnetic resonance angiography is usually negative because of the involvement of small blood vessels (arterioles). However, when the lacunar distribution of infarction is larger than expected, MRA can detect occlusion of a parent artery (e.g., middle cerebral artery occlusion causing infarction in the distribution of the lenticulostriate perforators)

Acute Head Trauma

Presenting Signs and Symptoms

Focal neurologic deficits (caused by intracerebral and extracerebral hematomas)

Generalized or focal cerebral edema that may lead to symptoms of herniation (through tentorium or foramen magnum)

Concussion (post-traumatic loss of consciousness)

Approach to Diagnostic Imaging

▶ 1. **Computed tomography**
  - ▶ Preferred study to detect skull fracture, *acute* intraparenchymal bleeding, and extra-axial hemorrhage (acute subdural and epidural hematoma)
  - ▶ The use of wider windows improves the ability of CT images to delineate isodense extracerebral hematoma. Ventricular shift and sulcal effacement are also subtle findings that should make one suspicious of the presence of an isodense subdural hematoma

▶ 2. **Magnetic resonance imaging**
  - ▶ Indicated only in those unusual cases in which CT has failed to detect an abnormality in the presence of strong clinical suspicion of intracranial hemorrhage (primarily in the posterior fossa or high on the convexity, areas in which CT may be limited because of overlying bone)
  - ▶ Particularly valuable in *subacute* and *chronic* phases of head trauma to define temporal and inferior frontal lobe hemorrhagic contusion and edema as well as shear injuries (subtle hemorrhage seen as low signal on gradient echo images) at the grey-white junctions and posterior corpus callosum

Note: There is *no* indication for plain skull radiography in this condition. The mere detection of a skull fracture generally has little effect on subsequent medical or surgical management. In addition, skull fractures usually are easily recognizable on CT, which can also delineate any accompanying abnormality in the underlying brain.

Epidural Hematoma

Presenting Signs and Symptoms

Symptoms developing within minutes or hours after injury (often after a lucid interval of relative neurologic normalcy)

Increasing headache, deterioration of consciousness, motor dysfunction, and pupillary changes indicate an *emergency* situation

Common Cause

Trauma (causing arterial laceration in the epidural space)

Approach to Diagnostic Imaging

▶ I. Computed tomography
  ▶ Preferred study for demonstrating the characteristic appearance of a collection of hyperintense hemorrhage convex to the brain that is located in the temporal region (middle meningeal artery) and often associated with a skull fracture

Note: There is *no* indication for plain skull radiographs in this condition.

Acute Subdural Hematoma

Presenting Signs and Symptoms

Progressive neurologic deterioration with signs of herniation

Deepening coma

Spastic hemiplegia with hyperreflexia

Common Cause

Head trauma

Approach to Diagnostic Imaging

▶ 1. **Computed tomography**
  - ▶ Preferred study for detection of the characteristically hyperintense, medially concave, lenticular extra-axial collection of blood in the subdural space

 Caveat: Thin subdural hematomas may be obscured by overlying bone (especially if they are located high on the convexity). Subfrontal or subtemporal hematomas may be difficult to detect on axial views and may require coronal reformatting or direct coronal imaging.

▶ 2. **Magnetic resonance imaging**
  - ▶ Although not as sensitive for detecting acute bleeding, the ability of MRI to directly obtain coronal images may be of value if CT fails to demonstrate a subdural hematoma in the face of strongly suggestive clinical findings

Note: There is *no* indication for plain skull films in this clinical setting.

Chronic Subdural Hematoma

Presenting Signs and Symptoms

History of head trauma (2–4 weeks or more prior to clinical presentation) that may have been relatively trivial and forgotten

Increasing headache

Fluctuating drowsiness or confusion

Mild-to-moderate hemiparesis

Typically occurs in alcoholics and patients older than the age of 50

Common Cause

Head trauma

Approach to Diagnostic Imaging

▶ I. **Magnetic resonance imaging**
  - ▶ Preferred study for detecting hemorrhages more than a few days old as hyperintense lesions on both T1- and T2-weighted images
  - ▶ Of particular value in detecting hemorrhages in the posterior fossa and high on the convexity (difficult areas for CT because of bone artifacts)
  - ▶ Clearly defines secondary findings such as brain contusion or hematoma, axonal shear injury at the grey-white junction and posterior corpus callosum, occipital infarction secondary to prior transtentorial herniation, and communicating hydrocephalus and atrophy

Notes: Unlike CT scans, on which hemorrhage becomes isodense after several weeks and thus may be impossible to recognize, on MRI hemorrhage may remain hyperintense and easily detectable for a year or more.

There is *no* indication for plain skull radiographs in this clinical situation.

Blow-Out Fracture of the Orbit

Presenting Signs and Symptoms

History of trauma
Extraocular eye movement abnormality

Approach to Diagnostic Imaging

▶ 1. **Plain radiograph (Waters view)**
   ▶ Preferred screening study to show bony discontinuity and the presence of a soft-tissue mass in the superior aspect of the maxillary antrum

▶ 2. **Computed tomography (axial and coronal scans)**
   ▶ Definitive study to show the fracture and the extent of herniation of orbital tissues through the defect into the superior aspect of the maxillary antrum

---

Note: If a blow-out fracture is suspected clinically, CT can be the initial imaging procedure (omitting plain radiography).

Facial Fracture

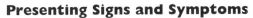

Presenting Signs and Symptoms

Facial swelling and ecchymoses

Approach to Diagnostic Imaging

▶ 1. **Plain radiograph**
   - ▶ Preferred screening study to demonstrate facial fractures (most commonly involve the nose, zygomatic arches, lateral walls of the maxillary antra, and floor of the orbit)

▶ 2. **Computed tomography**
   - ▶ Indicated if plain radiographs demonstrate a complex fracture that must be defined or suggests a blow-out fracture of the floor of the orbit
   - ▶ Both axial *and* coronal scans are usually required for full evaluation

Temporal Bone Fracture

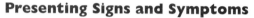

Presenting Signs and Symptoms

Various symptoms depending on the site of the fracture
(hearing loss, vertigo, nystagmus, facial paralysis)
Hemorrhage behind the tympanic membrane

Common Cause

Trauma

Approach to Diagnostic Imaging

▶ I. Computed tomography

> ▶ In addition to demonstrating the lucent fracture
> line (often requires thin cuts), CT may show sec-
> ondary signs of fracture such as fluid within the
> mastoid air cells or tympanic cavity, intracranial
> gas or gas within the temporomandibular joint,
> and disruption of the ossicular chain

Cervical Spine Trauma

Approach to Diagnostic Imaging

▶ 1. **Plain skeletal radiograph**
  - ▶ Preferred initial screening procedure quickly and inexpensively obtained, without significant disruption of other resuscitation efforts

---

> **Note:** Cross-table lateral view is generally obtained first, to avoid moving a patient who might have a cervical fracture; if it appears normal, additional films (including flexion and extension views) may be obtained.

 Caveat: It is *absolutely imperative* that all 7 cervical vertebral bodies be seen to avoid missing lower cervical spine fracture obscured by the shoulders. If the entire cervical spine is not seen, the film must be repeated with the shoulders lowered.

▶ 2. **Computed tomography**
  - ▶ Indicated if plain skeletal radiographs are equivocal or show a complex fracture of the cervical spine (especially involving the foramen transversarium, housing the vertebral artery that may be compromised by cervical trauma)
  - ▶ May be required in a trauma victim whose plain films are negative but who has substantial neck pain or neurologic deficits

▶ 3. **Magnetic resonance imaging**
  - ▶ Best procedure for detecting cord contusion and edema (and its sequela, myelomalacia), herniated disk, canal compromise, or epidural hematoma complicating trauma to the cervical spine

---

> **Note:** In a patient with suspected nerve root avulsion, either CT myelography or MRI can confirm the diagnosis.

Acromegaly/Gigantism

Presenting Signs and Symptoms

Soft tissue and bony overgrowth (increased size of the hand, foot, jaw, and cranium)

Coarsening of facial features

Peripheral neuropathies

Headache

Impaired glucose tolerance

Common Cause

Pituitary adenoma (excessive secretion of growth hormone)

Approach to Diagnostic Imaging

▶ I. **Magnetic resonance imaging**
  - ▶ Preferred study for detecting and defining the extent of the underlying pituitary tumor (superb sensitivity and multiplanar capability)
  - ▶ Permits clear distinction of the sphenoid sinus and the position of the carotid artery for surgical planning
  - ▶ If an aneurysm is suspected on MR imaging, MR angiography is obtained

---

Note: There is *no* indication for plain radiographs of the sella in this condition.

Diabetes Insipidus

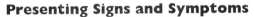

Presenting Signs and Symptoms

Excretion of excessive quantities of urine (polyuria) that is very dilute but otherwise normal

Excessive thirst (polydipsia)

Dehydration and hypovolemia (develops rapidly if urinary losses are not continuously replaced)

Common Causes

PRIMARY (IDIOPATHIC)

Marked decrease in hypothalamic nuclei of neurohypophyseal system and deficient production of vasopressin (antidiuretic hormone)

SECONDARY (ACQUIRED)

Hypophysectomy

Cranial injury (especially basal skull fracture)

Suprasellar and intrasellar neoplasm (primary or metastatic)

Histiocytosis X

Granulomatous disease (tuberculosis, sarcoidosis)

Vascular lesion (aneurysm, thrombosis)

Infection (encephalitis, meningitis)

Approach to Diagnostic Imaging

▶ I. **Magnetic resonance imaging**

▶ Preferred study for demonstrating any underlying lesion of the hypothalamus, pituitary gland, or pituitary stalk (superb sensitivity, multiplanar capability)

Note: High-resolution, thin-section study is required; contrast enhancement improves sensitivity.

Galactorrhea/Amenorrhea

Presenting Signs and Symptoms

WOMEN

Galactorrhea

Menstrual disturbances

Infertility

Symptoms of estrogen deficiency (hot flashes, dyspareunia)

MEN

Loss of libido and potency

Infertility (occasional galactorrhea or gynecomastia)

Common Causes

Prolactinoma of pituitary gland

Drugs (phenothiazines, antihypertensives)

Primary hypothyroidism

Hypothalamic/pituitary stalk disease

Approach to Diagnostic Imaging

▶ 1. **Magnetic resonance imaging**

▶ Preferred study for demonstrating the prolactin-secreting pituitary microadenoma (usually < 1 cm) that is the underlying cause in about half of the cases

▶ Requires thin-section imaging in both the coronal and sagittal planes

---

Note: There is *no* indication for plain films of the sella in this condition.

Hypopituitarism

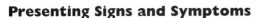

Presenting Signs and Symptoms

Variable depending on which specific pituitary hormones are deficient (gonadotropins, growth hormone, thyroid-stimulating hormone, and adrenocorticotrophic hormone)

Common Causes

PITUITARY LESION

Tumor (adenoma, craniopharyngioma)
Infarction or ischemic necrosis
Inflammatory or infiltrative process (e.g., sarcoidosis)
Iatrogenic (irradiation or surgical removal)

HYPOTHALAMIC LESION

Tumor
Inflammation
Trauma

Approach to Diagnostic Imaging

▶ I. **Magnetic resonance imaging**
  ▶ Preferred study because of its superb sensitivity and ability to directly image the sella and parasellar regions in multiple planes

---

Note: There is *no* indication for plain films of the sella in this condition.

Herniated Nucleus Pulposus

Presenting Signs and Symptoms

Pain in the distribution of compressed nerve roots (may be sudden and severe or more insidious)

Pain increased by movement or Valsalva maneuver

Paresthesias or numbness in the sensory distribution of the affected roots

Reduced or absent deep tendon reflexes in the distribution of involved nerve roots

Weakness and eventual atrophy of muscles supplied by affected nerves

Positive straight leg raising test (lumbosacral region)

Urinary incontinence or retention (from loss of sphincter function in lumbosacral involvement)

Most common in the lower lumbosacral and lower cervical regions

Common Cause

Degenerative disk disease

Approach to Diagnostic Imaging

▶ I. **Magnetic resonance imaging**
  - ▶ Most sensitive study for demonstrating bulging, protrusion, extrusion, or free fragmentation of disk material as well as impingement on the spinal cord and individual spinal nerve roots
  - ▶ Can show degeneration of the disk as loss of signal on T2-weighted images (although this may be of little clinical importance)
  - ▶ Can distinguish among canal stenosis, degenerative facet overgrowth, and herniated disk
  - ▶ Permits routine visualization of conus medullaris

▶ **2. Computed tomography**
  ▶ Useful for detecting herniated disk and canal steno-
    sis, but limited by single imaging plane, poor
    visualization of the conus without intrathecal
    contrast material, and poor assessment of the
    postoperative spine

 Caveat: *Plain radiographs* of the spine
  may demonstrate disk space narrowing and
  hypertrophic spurring. However, they do
  not give any indication of whether there is
  critical impingement on the vertebral canal
  or nerve roots and, therefore, are of little
  value when MRI or CT is used.

  Myelography is *not* indicated in the evaluation of disease involving the intervertebral
  disks.

Sciatica

Presenting Signs and Symptoms

Pain radiating down one or both buttocks and the posterior aspect of the leg(s) to below the knee (the distribution of the sciatic nerve)

Common Causes

Peripheral nerve root compression (intervertebral disk protrusion or intraspinal tumor)

Compression within the spinal canal or intervertebral foramen (tumor, osteoarthritis, spondylolisthesis)

Approach to Diagnostic Imaging

▶ 1. **Magnetic resonance imaging**
   - ▶ Most sensitive study for demonstrating bulging, protrusion, extrusion, or free fragmentation of disk material, as well as impingement on the spinal cord, conus, and individual nerve roots

▶ 2. **Computed tomography**
   - ▶ CT is still also valuable for detecting herniated disk and bony foraminal or canal stenosis
   - ▶ Disadvantages are poor visualization of the conus; inability to distinguish herniated disk from scar in the postoperative spine; essentially single axial-plane imaging; and radiation dose

 Caveat: *Plain spinal radiographs* may demonstrate disk space narrowing and hypertrophic spurring. However, they do not give any indication of whether there is critical impingement on the spinal cord or nerve roots.

Myelography is not indicated in the evaluation of sciatica and generally is not required if MRI or CT has been performed.

Scoliosis

Presenting Signs and Symptoms

Structural lateral curvature of the spine that may be suspected when one shoulder appears higher than the other or if clothes do not hang straight

Fatigue in the lumbar region after prolonged sitting or standing that may be associated with muscular backaches

Common Causes

Idiopathic

Vertebral anomaly

Hydromyelia and dysraphic states

Approach to Diagnostic Imaging

▶ **1. Plain spinal radiograph**
  ▸ Demonstrates the site and severity of the curvature (typically convex to the right in the thoracic area and to the left in the lumbar area so that the right shoulder is higher than the left)

▶ **2. Magnetic resonance imaging**
  ▸ Indicated to exclude an intraspinal abnormality if scoliosis is severe or has an early age of onset, or if plain radiographs show a vertebral anomaly

---

Note: MRI is required to detect series anomalies such as tethered cord that must be addressed before the spine undergoes mechanical straightening. Coverage from the cervicomedullary junction to the sacral level is generally needed (T1-weighted images often are sufficient).

Spinal Stenosis

Presenting Signs and Symptoms

Pain in buttocks, thighs, or calves on walking, running, or climbing stairs, not relieved by standing still but by flexing the back, sitting, or lying down

Common Causes

Degenerative disease (hypertrophy of facets or ligamentum flavum, disk protrusion, postoperative scarring, synovial cyst)

Paget's disease

Achondroplasia

Trauma

Severe spondylolisthesis

Approach to Diagnostic Imaging

▶ 1. **Magnetic resonance imaging or computed tomography**
   - ▶ Both demonstrate bony and soft-tissue changes causing compression of thecal sac or spinal cord centrally, as well as encroachment of the nerve root in the neural foramen or lateral recess
   - ▶ Study of choice because of multiplanar capability and ability to better visualize the conus

    Caveat: *Plain spinal radiographs* may demonstrate disk space narrowing and hypertrophic spurring. However, they do not show whether there is critical impingement on the spinal cord or nerve roots. Disk space narrowing and vertebral body alignment are better defined using MRI.

   Myelography is not indicated in evaluation of disease involving the intervertebral disks or the spinal canal. Risk of epidural injection and severe discomfort are greatest in patients with spinal stenosis.

Failed Back Syndrome

Presenting Signs and Symptoms

No relief of neurologic symptoms after surgical procedure for herniated nucleus pulposus (occurs in the lumbar region in about 10–25% of patients)

Common Causes

Recurrent or residual disk
Scarring
Lateral or central canal stenosis
Adhesive arachnoiditis
Conus abnormality

Approach to Diagnostic Imaging

► I. **Magnetic resonance imaging**
  ► Most accurate technique for making the crucial distinction between recurrent/residual disk and scar
  ► Scar appears hyperintense to the annulus on T2-weighted scans (recurrent disk is hypointense) and enhances homogeneously after contrast administration (chronic disk herniation may have some peripheral enhancement because of surrounding granulation tissue)
  ► Must be analyzed carefully for canal stenosis, far-lateral herniated disc, and conus mass

Syringomyelia/ Hydromyelia

Presenting Signs and Symptoms

Spasticity and weakness of the lower extremities

Sensory defect (typically begins in the cervical region and often extends to a capelike defect over the shoulders and back)

Common Causes

Congenital (often associated with Chiari malformation and encephalocele)

Intramedullary tumor (if no associated Chiari I)

Trauma (post-traumatic syrinx or cystic myelomalacia)

Approach to Diagnostic Imaging

► I. **Magnetic resonance imaging**
  - ► Demonstrates the atrophic (chronic) or enlarged spinal cord with central cystic, haustrated cavity
  - ► Associated Chiari I malformation is common
  - ► Upper margin of the hydromyelia cavity is at the level of the pyramidal decussation (cephalad cervical cord)
  - ► If there is no Chiari malformation or the cystic central cord lesion does not respect the pyramidal decussation boundary and extends above the cervicomedullary junction, contrast infusion is indicated to detect an underlying spinal cord neoplasm (hemangioblastoma, ependymoma, astrocytoma)

Tethered Cord
(Low Conus)

Presenting Signs and Symptoms

Back pain
Dyesthesias
Neurogenic bladder
Spasticity
Congenital/developmental kyphoscoliosis

Approach to Diagnostic Imaging

▶ I. **Magnetic resonance imaging**
 ▶ Preferred study for showing the low-lying (below
  L2–L3 level), posteriorly tethered conus medullaris and thickened filum terminale that may ter-
  minate in a lipoma or dermoid

Note: MRI of the entire spine is generally performed
to evaluate for hydrosyringomyelia and any abnormality at the cervicomedullary junction.

Transverse Myelitis (Acute)

Presenting Signs and Symptoms

Sudden onset of local back pain followed by sensory symptoms and motor weakness ascending from the feet

Urinary retention and loss of bowel control

Common Causes

Unknown (may be related to a prior viral illness, vasculitis, or intravenous use of heroin or amphetamine)

Approach to Diagnostic Imaging

▶ I. **Magnetic resonance imaging**
- ▶ In addition to showing focal enlargement of the spinal cord, T2-weighted images demonstrate high signal throughout the region of involvement
- ▶ An acute lesion shows contrast enhancement

Note: The role of MRI is more to exclude treatable conditions such as unsuspected cord compression than to make a specific diagnosis.

Anosmia

Presenting Sign and Symptom

Loss of sense of smell

Common Causes

Head trauma (especially in young adults)
Viral infection (especially in older adults)
Chronic nasal obstruction (polyps)
Neoplasm (interfering with olfactory apparatus)
Granulomatous disease
Male hypogonadism (Kallmann's syndrome)

Approach to Diagnostic Imaging

▶ 1. **Computed tomography**
  ▸ Can detect a neoplasm or unsuspected fracture of the floor of the anterior cranial fossa
  ▸ Can demonstrate polyps or other neoplastic or granulomatous processes resulting in nasal obstruction

▶ 2. **Magnetic resonance imaging**
  ▸ Can detect a subfrontal mass (e.g., meningioma, metastasis or direct extension from squamous cell carcinoma, esthesioneuroblastoma)
  ▸ Used for planning prior to surgery or radiation therapy

Bell's Palsy

Presenting Signs and Symptoms

Unilateral facial paralysis (sudden onset)

Pain behind the ear (may precede facial weakness)

Widening of palpebral fissure (prevents closure of eye)

Common Causes

Unknown (presumably swelling of the facial nerve due to immune or viral disease with resultant ischemia and compression of the nerve as it passes through its narrow canal in the temporal bone)

Approach to Diagnostic Imaging

▶ I. Magnetic resonance imaging

 ▶ Indicated to exclude a mass or demyelinating lesion within or adjacent to the facial nerve (from its brain stem origin to the parotid gland) if symptoms are recurrent, prolonged, progressive, or associated with dysfunction of other cranial nerves

> **Note:** High-resolution axial and coronal imaging is required.

▶ Demonstrates contrast enhancement in almost 80% of patients with clinical Bell's palsy (most commonly in the labyrinthine segment and descending facial nerve canal) that may persist past the point of clinical improvement

> ▼ **Caveat:** Unfortunately, the side of enhancement may not always correlate with the clinical symptoms.

Cerebrospinal Fluid Leak

Presenting Signs and Symptoms

Leakage of cerebrospinal fluid (identified by its glucose content) from the nose (rhinorrhea) or ears (otorrhea)

Common Causes

Fracture with dural tear

Nose: Communication develops between the subarachnoid space and the paranasal sinuses

Ear: Communication develops between the subarachnoid space and the middle ear (in association with disruption of the tympanic membrane)

Approach to Diagnostic Imaging

▶ 1. **Radionuclide cisternography**
   ▶ Procedure of choice that is extremely sensitive in demonstrating tiny amounts of radionuclide in cotton pledgets placed in the nostrils or external ears

 Caveat: This technique is unsatisfactory for localizing the precise site of leakage.

▶ 2. **Computed tomography (CT cisternography)**
   ▶ Thin-section scanning is performed both before and after the intrathecal injection of nonionic, iodinated contrast material via lumbar puncture

Note: Delayed imaging may be required a few hours later to detect subtle leakage.

 Caveat: Cerebrospinal fluid leakage often cannot be detected even using both radionuclide and CT cisternography.

Multiple Sclerosis

Presenting Signs and Symptoms

Variety of focal neurologic dysfunctions characterized by erratic remissions and exacerbations

Paresthesias (extremity, trunk, or face)

Weakness or clumsiness of leg or hand

Visual disturbances (optic neuritis)

Abnormalities of gait and coordination

Common Causes

Unknown (possibly viral or immune related)

Increased risk in persons living in northern climates (e.g., northern United States, Canada, Scandinavia) before puberty

Approach to Diagnostic Imaging

▶ I. **Magnetic resonance imaging**

 ▶ Most sensitive study for detection of the scattered plaques of demyelination that are hyperintense to brain on T2-weighted images

  ▶ Greater specificity with lesions involving the inferior corpus callosum, white matter about the temporal horn, middle cerebral peduncle, and discrete lesions in the pons or the posterior column of the cervical portion of the spinal cord

  ▶ Lesions involving the optic nerve or chiasm are difficult to detect without contrast enhancement and fat suppression

  ▼ **Caveat:** CT should *not* be requested because it is generally normal during the early stages of the disease.

Normal Pressure Hydrocephalus

Presenting Signs and Symptoms

Dementia
Gait disturbance
Urinary incontinence

Common Causes

Previous surface inflammation of the brain due to sub-arachnoid hemorrhage or diffuse meningitis (postulated to cause scarring of arachnoid villi over brain convexities where cerebrospinal fluid absorption usually occurs)

Approach to Diagnostic Imaging

▶ 1. **Magnetic resonance imaging**
- ▶ Demonstrates the dilated ventricular system (out of proportion to the degree of sulcal prominence) and can exclude the various causes of noncommunicating obstructive hydrocephalus
- ▶ Sagittal scans show thinning of the corpus callosum and decreased mamillopontine distance as well as accentuation of the signal void in the aqueduct of Sylvius and the posterior part of the third ventricle

▶ 2. **Radionuclide cisternography**
- ▶ Demonstrates "reflux" of radionuclide into the lateral ventricles and delayed clearance of isotope from the lateral ventricles and cerebral convexities ("stasis")

Obstructive Hydrocephalus

Presenting Signs and Symptoms

Headache

Nausea and vomiting

Drowsiness

Diplopia, blurred vision

Papilledema

Palsy of sixth cranial nerve

Pupillary dilatation, coma, decerebrate posturing, abnormal respirations, systemic hypertension, and bradycardia (may develop if increased intracranial pressure is not controlled)

Common Sites of Obstruction and Causes

Foramen of Monro
    Neoplasm

Posterior fossa (aqueduct of Sylvius, fourth ventricle, foramen of Luschka/Magendie)
    Congenital stenosis
    Neoplasm
    Cerebellar infarction/hematoma
    Posterior fossa extra-axial and Dandy-Walker cyst

Subarachnoid spaces
    Meningitis
    Sarcoidosis
    Carcinomatosis
    Subarachnoid hemorrhage

Other
    Venous thrombosis
    Choroid plexus papilloma

Approach to Diagnostic Imaging

▶ I. **Magnetic resonance imaging**
  - ▶ Not only shows the dilated ventricular system but also may demonstrate the underlying cause of obstruction to the flow of cerebrospinal fluid in the noncommunicating type of hydrocephalus
  - ▶ Excellent for imaging lesions of the posterior fossa. Contrast enhancement may assist in distinguishing a congenital posterior fossa cyst from an enhancing cystic neoplasm.

Optic Neuritis

Presenting Signs and Symptoms

Visual loss (ranging from a small central or paracentral scotoma to complete blindness) that is usually unilateral

Depressed direct pupillary light reflex

Common Causes

Multiple sclerosis
Viral illness
Ischemia (e.g., temporal arteritis)
Meningitis
Syphilis
Sarcoidosis
Systemic lupus erythematosus

Approach to Diagnostic Imaging

▶ I. **Magnetic resonance imaging**

  ▶ In addition to showing enlargement and contrast enhancement of the optic nerve (also seen on CT), MRI is the preferred study because it is the best screening test for detecting the characteristic white matter demyelination changes of multiple sclerosis (the most common cause of optic neuritis in adults)

  ▶ To best visualize enhancement in the optic nerves, fat suppression is required

Orbital Pseudotumor

Presenting Signs and Symptoms

Acute onset of painful proptosis, chemosis, and decreased motility of the extraocular muscles

Usually unilateral (85%) and exquisitely sensitive to steroids

Common Causes

Idiopathic inflammatory reaction (most likely autoimmune, but may be associated with such systemic diseases as Wegener's granulomatosis, lymphoma, fibrosing mediastinitis, thyroiditis, cholangitis, and vasculitis)

Approach to Diagnostic Imaging

▶ I. Computed tomography
  ▶ The confusing spectrum of findings includes a discrete soft-tissue mass within the retrobulbar fat, and thickening and contrast enhancement of the extraocular muscles, sclera, optic nerve, and lacrimal gland

---

Note: It may be difficult to distinguish from thyroid ophthalmopathy, which involves inferior > medial > superior rectus muscles.

Progressive Multifocal Leukoencephalopathy

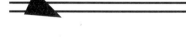

Presenting Signs and Symptoms

Hemiparesis, seizures, blindness, intellectual dysfunction, and cerebellar or brainstem dysfunction that is relentlessly progressive (death within 6 months)

Common Causes

Papovavirus (universal childhood infection that is reactivated in the immunosuppressed patient with AIDS, leukemia, or lymphoma)

Approach to Diagnostic Imaging

▶ I. Magnetic resonance imaging
  ▶ Demonstrates asymmetric focal white matter lesions in both the cerebrum and cerebellum that typically show no edema, mass effect, or contrast enhancement (blood-brain barrier remains intact)

Note: CT is not as effective in showing this primarily white matter process.

Pseudotumor Cerebri

Presenting Signs and Symptoms

Headache and papilledema (increased intracranial pressure) in an otherwise apparently healthy patient

Partial or complete monocular visual loss in 5% (usually intact visual acuity and central visual fields)

Common Causes

Unknown (spontaneous onset and eventual disappearance; patients often overweight)

In children, may follow withdrawal of steroid therapy or excessive ingestion of vitamin A or tetracycline

Risk Factors

Obesity

Endocrine dysfunction

Sinovenous thrombosis

Hematologic disorders

Increased cerebrospinal fluid protein

Meningitis

Approach to Diagnostic Imaging

▶ I. **Magnetic resonance imaging or computed tomography**
   ▶ To exclude a space-occupying mass or venous occlusion causing increased intracranial pressure

Radiation Necrosis

Presenting Signs and Symptoms

Progression of neurologic deficit (some patients exhibit no new symptoms)

Approach to Diagnostic Imaging

▶ I. **Magnetic resonance imaging**
  - ▶ Imaging modality of choice for demonstrating both the acute and delayed effects of therapeutic radiation

> **Note:** MRI is substantially more sensitive than CT for detecting the predominantly white matter alterations caused by radiation necrosis and radiation injury.

▶ 2. **Positron emission tomography**
  - ▶ In the absence of clinical or radiographic criteria, PET scanning using ^{18}F-deoxyglucose (FDG) as a marker of cellular metabolism is the best technique for distinguishing recurrent or residual tumor (hypermetabolic) from areas of radiation necrosis (hypometabolic)

HEAD AND NECK

William Dillon

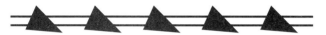

Endocrine Disorders
Hyperparathyroidism
Hyperthyroidism
Hypercalcemia
Hypothyroidism (Myxedema)

Masses
Cancer of the Larynx
Cancer of the Pharynx
Thyroid Mass
Cancer of the Thyroid
Salivary Gland (Parotid) Neoplasm
Occult Primary with Positive Lymphadenopathy

Other
Sinusitis
Cranial Neuropathy
Internal Disk Derangement of Temporomandibular Joint

Hyperparathyroidism

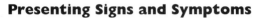

Presenting Signs and Symptoms

May be asymptomatic (50%)

Renal disease (nephrolithiasis and nephrocalcinosis)

Peripheral neuromuscular disease (proximal muscle weakness, fatiguability, atrophy)

Gastrointestinal disease (peptic ulcers, pancreatitis)

Neuropsychiatric dysfunction

Common Causes

PRIMARY

Parathyroid adenoma (89%)

Parathyroid hyperplasia (10%)

Parathyroid carcinoma (1%)

SECONDARY

Chronic renal failure

PARANEOPLASTIC SYNDROMES

Bronchogenic and renal cell carcinoma

Approach to Diagnostic Imaging

▶ I. **Plain skeletal radiograph (hands and other skeletal sites)**

▶ May demonstrate characteristic subperiosteal resorption of radial aspect of the middle phalanges of the hand, resorption of phalangeal tufts, erosion of distal clavicles, sclerotic stripes in vertebral bodies ("rugby jersey" spine), and punched-out lesions in the skull ("salt-and-pepper" appearance)

> **Note:** Although once routinely obtained, there is *no* need for a "metabolic bone survey" (including the long bones and spine), because the yield of positive findings is extremely low and a positive finding rarely affects treatment. *If any* radiographic study is required, plain films of the hands should suffice.

Detection of Parathyroid Gland Abnormality

▶ 1. **Ultrasound**
  - ▸ Preferred screening technique that can detect 80–85% of abnormal parathyroid glands located near the thyroid
  - ▸ Parathyroid carcinomas tend to have a more heterogeneous internal architecture than adenomas

▶ 2. **Computed tomography or magnetic resonance imaging**
  - ▸ Generally required to detect abnormal parathyroid tissue at ectopic sites such as the thymus (10–15%), the posterior mediastinum (5%), those within the carotid sheath, and those that are retroesophageal or parapharyngeal

▶ 3. **Technetium-thallium radionuclide subtraction imaging**
  - ▸ Screening technique for detecting parathyroid adenomas (sensitivity 75%; specificity 90%), which is based on the fact that thyroid tissue concentrates both thallium and technetium, whereas a parathyroid adenoma picks up only radioactive thallium (and appears as a residual focus of activity when the technetium image is subtracted from the thallium image)

 Caveat: **False-positive results can result from thallium uptake in thyroid nodules, sarcoid lymph nodes, or metastases to the neck.**

Hyperthyroidism

Presenting Signs and Symptoms

Goiter
Weight loss with increased appetite
Warm, moist skin
Heat intolerance
Tremor
Irritability and insomnia
Palpitations and tachycardia
Muscle weakness
Exophthalmos
Frequent bowel movements
Thyroid storm (thyrotoxicosis)
Proptosis

Common Causes

Graves' disease (toxic diffuse goiter)
Toxic multinodular goiter (Plummer's disease)
Toxic adenoma
Thyroiditis (subacute or painless)
Thyrotoxicosis factitia (ingestion of thyroid hormone tablets)

Approach to Diagnostic Imaging

 Caveat: The diagnosis of hyperthyroidism is made clinically by routine thyroid hormone determinations, and there usually is no need for routine imaging studies.

▶ I. **Radionuclide thyroid scan**
  ▶ Indicated to distinguish Graves' disease from multinodular goiter or a single toxic adenoma

▶ **2. Radioactive iodine uptake**
  - ▸ Although long used to measure thyroid function, this test has been supplanted by radioimmunoassay techniques and the development of accurate methods to measure serum levels of thyroid hormones and stimulating factors
  - ▸ Radioactive iodine uptake currently is performed primarily for differentiating Graves' disease (high uptake) from subacute or painless thyroiditis (low uptake), and in assisting in the calculation of the dose of radioactive iodine for the treatment of Graves' disease

▶ **3. Computed tomography**
  - ▸ CT scans of the orbits may be required in cases of Graves' ophthalmography, in which diffuse enlargement of the extraocular muscles results in proptosis, chemosis, and occasionally visual loss from compression of the optic nerve

Hypercalcemia

Presenting Signs and Symptoms

Usually asymptomatic (discovered incidentally during routine laboratory screening)

Constipation, anorexia, nausea and vomiting, abdominal pain, adynamic ileus

Nephrolithiasis (or urolithiasis) and nephrocalcinosis; polyuria, nocturia, and polydipsia; renal failure

Skeletal muscular weakness

Emotional lability, confusion, delirium, psychosis, stupor, coma

Common Causes

Hyperparathyroidism (primary)

Chronic renal failure (secondary hyperparathyroidism)

Excessive gastrointestinal absorption and/or intake (milk-alkali syndrome, vitamin D intoxication, sarcoidosis)

Endocrine dysfunction (hypothyroidism, Addison's disease)

Skeletal metastases/myeloma

Humoral hypercalcemia of malignancy (no bone metastases)

Immobilization

Drug therapy (thiazides, lithium, aluminum-containing antacids)

Approach to Diagnostic Imaging

Clinical assessment is necessary to direct the imaging approach

Radiographs of the hands, pelvis, and spine are useful for evaluating hyperparathyroidism (hands) or metastasis or myeloma (pelvis, spine)

Note: See individual underlying disorders.

Hypothyroidism (Myxedema)

Presenting Signs and Symptoms

Weight gain
Dull facial expression with hoarse voice and slow speech
Periorbital swelling and drooping eyelids
Cold intolerance
Sluggishness
Sparse, coarse, dry hair
Coarse, dry, scaly skin
Constipation

Common Causes

Dietary iodine deficiency (endemic goiter)
Chronic thyroiditis (Hashimoto's disease)
Treated hyperthyroidism (radioactive iodine or surgery)
Failure of hypothalamic-pituitary axis (deficient secretion of thyrotropin-releasing hormone or thyroid-stimulating hormone)

Approach to Diagnostic Imaging

 Caveat: The diagnosis of hypothyroidism is made clinically by routine thyroid hormone determinations, and there usually is no need for routine imaging studies.

Note: Although long used to measure thyroid function, radionuclide iodine uptake has been supplanted by radioimmunoassay techniques and the development of accurate methods to measure serum levels of thyroid hormones and stimulating factors.

Cancer of the Larynx

Presenting Signs and Symptoms

Neck mass in smoker older than 40 years (male > female)

Hoarseness

Stridor

Common Sites

True vocal cord

Supraglottic

Approach to Diagnostic Imaging

▶ 1. **Computed tomography**
   - ▶ Thin-section CT is the best modality for demonstrating the extent of disease

▶ 2. **Magnetic resonance imaging**
   - ▶ Preferred modality for evaluating the mucosa and cartilages
   - ▶ Superior to CT for defining the infraglottic spread of disease

    Caveat: Because postbiopsy changes may simulate occult carcinoma, **CT** and **MRI** should be performed before biopsy if possible.

Cancer of the Pharynx

Presenting Signs and Symptoms

Neck mass in smoker older than 40 years of age (male > female)

Referred otalgia (ear pain)

Chronic sore throat

Cranial nerve palsy

Decreased hearing (due to serous effusion within ear)

Common Sites

Tongue, floor of mouth, tonsil, oropharynx, base of tongue, larynx, pyriform sinus (nasopharynx is less common)

Approach to Diagnostic Imaging

▶ 1. **Magnetic resonance imaging**
  - ▶ Preferred modality for evaluating the pharyngeal mucosa and other sites where occult disease may reside
  - ▶ Superior technique for defining intracranial spread of disease and involvement of the carotid artery

▶ 2. **Computed tomography**
  - ▶ High-speed CT may permit evaluation of the site of the neck mass and cervical adenopathy

---

Note: Contrast infusion is required to differentiate lymph nodes from vessels.

 Caveat: Because postbiopsy changes may simulate occult carcinoma, **MRI and CT should be performed before biopsy if possible.**

Thyroid Mass

Common Causes

Diffuse or nodular goiter
Thyroiditis
Abscess
Cyst
Neoplasm (adenoma, carcinoma, metastases, lymphoma)

Approach to Diagnostic Imaging

▶ I. **Radionuclide thyroid scan**

▶ Preferred screening procedure for demonstrating hypofunctioning (cold) nodules (10–20% representing carcinoma) and hyperfunctioning (hot) nodules (rarely malignant)

 Caveat: Although radionuclide scanning can detect thyroid nodules, it cannot discriminate benign from malignant processes.

► **2. Ultrasound**
  - ► Primarily indicated to determine whether a non-functioning thyroid mass detected on a radionuclide scan is cystic or solid (purely cystic or hyperechoic masses are rarely malignant)
  - ► Of special value in patients in whom exogenous iodine contamination from prior contrast studies precludes a radionuclide scan

 Caveat: As with radionuclide scanning, ultrasound cannot determine whether a hypoechoic mass is benign or malignant.

Note: CT and MRI are primarily used to demonstrate a substernal thyroid that cannot be detected by ultrasound because of overlying bone.

Cancer of the Thyroid

Presenting Signs and Symptoms

Asymptomatic (felt by the patient or detected on physical examination)

Recurrent laryngeal palsy

Hoarseness

Metastasis to cervical nodes or remote sites

Approach to Diagnostic Imaging

▶ **1. Radionuclide thyroid scan**
   ▶ Single hypofunctioning (cold) nodule has a 10–20% chance of being malignant

---

Note: A history of neck irradiation, especially in childhood, increases the risk of malignancy by 5–10 times.

▶ **2. Ultrasound**
   ▶ Primarily indicated to determine whether a nonfunctioning thyroid mass detected on a radionuclide scan is cystic or solid (purely cystic or hyperechoic masses are rarely malignant)
   ▶ Of special value in patients in whom exogenous iodine contamination from prior contrast studies precludes a radionuclide scan

 Caveat: Because neither radionuclide scans nor ultrasound (and neither CT nor MRI) can definitely determine whether a nonfunctioning, hypoechoic mass is benign or malignant, aspiration biopsy is required in every suspicious case.

Note: Regression of nodule size following thyroid hormone therapy is a sign of a benign nodule.

Staging

▶ 1. **Computed tomography or magnetic resonance imaging**

- ▸ Procedures of choice to demonstrate involvement of adjacent muscles, larynx, esophagus, and other neck structures by a large invasive tumor
- ▸ MRI may better demonstrate the relationship of the carotid vessels to the tumor; CT is easier for imaging the chest and mediastinum

▶ 2. **Whole-body radionuclide scan (^{131}I)**

- ▸ Effectively demonstrates thyroid metastases following thyroidectomy for *papillary* carcinoma

 Caveat: This technique is of no value for medullary or anaplastic carcinoma because these tumors do not take up iodine.

Detecting Recurrences

▶ 1. **Magnetic resonance imaging**

- ▸ Modality of choice for detecting recurrent tumor, which appears as an area of high-signal intensity on T2-weighted images

---

Note: On T2-weighted images, fibrosis has low-signal intensity, which is less than or equal to adjacent muscle.

▶ 2. **Whole-body radionuclide scan (^{131}I)**

- ▸ Focal activity in the lungs, skeleton, or neck remote from the thyroid bed is evidence of recurrence

---

Note: Uptake of radionuclide in the thyroid bed often represents residual thyroid tissue; uptake in the stomach, bowel, bladder, and salivary glands reflects physiologic traces of normal iodine distribution; and uptake in the breast also may be a normal finding.

Salivary Gland (Parotid) Neoplasm

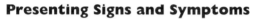

Presenting Signs and Symptoms

Palpable mass (slightly tender or nontender)
Facial palsy
Parapharyngeal mass

If *benign cyst,* tends to develop quickly over several days, may be tender if infected, and often has a history of prior recurrent episodes

If *benign tumor,* slow-growing, painless, nontender, and mobile

If *malignant tumor,* tends to enlarge rapidly over several weeks and be slightly painful and minimally tender, hard and fixed on palpation, and often associated with facial nerve paralysis

Approach to Diagnostic Imaging

▶ I. **Computed tomography or magnetic resonance imaging**

▶ Preferred studies for identifying the presence of a mass or multiple masses; its location within the gland and its position relative to the facial nerve; whether the mass is smoothly marginated or infiltrating and necrotic, cystic, or solid; and whether the mass is confined to the gland or has extended outside the gland capsule into the upper neck and skull base

▶ CT is superior to MRI for detecting an underlying calcified stone

▶ MRI is superior to CT for sharply outlining the margins of the mass (what seems on CT to be a vague fullness may appear as a discrete mass on MRI; what appears as several different masses on CT may be shown to be a highly lobulated solitary mass on MRI)

 Caveat: The distinction between a benign and a malignant mass often cannot be made purely on the basis of **CT** or **MRI**. However, when combined with clinical findings, an accuracy rate of about 90% can be achieved.

Note: Fine-needle biopsy, often performed under CT guidance, can provide a precise pathologic diagnosis in more than 90% of cases.

Occult Primary with Positive Lymphadenopathy

Presenting Sign and Symptom

Neck mass in a smoker older than 40 years (male > female)

Common Causes

Squamous carcinoma of the pharynx, pyriform sinus, nasopharynx, or base of the tongue

Approach to Diagnostic Imaging

▶ **1. Magnetic resonance imaging**
- ▶ Preferred imaging modality for evaluating the pharyngeal mucosa and other sites where the occult malignancy may reside

▶ **2. Computed tomography**
- ▶ High-speed studies may detect the site of an occult carcinoma in about 25% of cases (thus permitting directed biopsy by endoscopy)

 Caveat: Because postbiopsy changes may simulate occult carcinoma, MRI and CT should be performed before biopsy if possible.

Sinusitis

Presenting Signs and Symptoms

Pain, tenderness, and swelling over the involved sinus
Fever and chills (suggests extension of infection beyond the sinuses)

Predisposing Factors

Recent acute viral upper respiratory infection
Dental infection

Approach to Diagnostic Imaging

► 1. **Plain radiograph (sinus)**
   ► Limited role in the assessment of sinus disease; preferred screening technique that may demonstrate air-fluid levels in *acute* sinusitis

► 2. **Computed tomography**
   ► Procedure of choice for exquisitely defining the sinonasal anatomy; may be best alternative to plain radiography in patients with suspected chronic sinusitis or in cases of suspected complications such as mucocele or osteomyelitis

► 3. **Magnetic resonance imaging**
   ► Indicated for suspected neoplasm underlying sinusitis or in patients with intracranial disease or neurologic symptoms
   ► May be the best modality for detecting and characterizing a mucocele
   ► Contrast MRI is the best technique for detecting subdural or epidural empyema

 Caveat: MRI should be restricted to assessing complications of sinusitis and not used as a screening examination.

Cranial Neuropathy

Common Causes

Neoplasm (primary of perineural spread)
Infection (viral or bacterial)
Radiation therapy

Approach to Diagnostic Imaging

▶ 1. **Magnetic resonance imaging**
  ▶ Study of choice for assessing cranial neuropathy of undetermined cause

Note: This study should be performed using contrast-enhanced, fat-saturated scans perpendicular to the course of the affected cranial nerve.

 Caveat: MR scans must examine the entire course of the nerve, from its origin in the brain stem to its distal ramifications.

▶ 2. **Computed tomography**
  ▶ Less sensitive than MRI for detecting early spread of carcinoma along cranial nerves

Note: CT should be performed using thin sections oriented to the appropriate plane of section and perpendicular to the involved nerve.

Specific Cranial Nerves

TRIGEMINAL NEUROPATHY (NOT TIC DOULOUREUX)

Most commonly due to a cerebellopontine angle mass or to perineural spread of tumor from the oral cavity or the head and neck

FACIAL PALSY

Most common cause of Bell's palsy

Does not require imaging unless facial function is slow to return or there is some other complicating factor (pain, dysfunction of other cranial nerves, parotid mass)

Must exclude parotid malignancy and temporal bone tumors (hemangioma, cholesteatoma, neurinoma)

Note: MRI is the imaging study of choice for the brainstem and parotid gland; CT may be useful for evaluating the temporal bone.

LOWER CRANIAL NERVES (9–12)

Most commonly due to a tumor at the skull base, which is best demonstrated by MRI

Differential diagnosis includes paraganglioma, meningioma, metastasis, and primary skull base tumor (e.g., chondrosarcoma)

THIRD CRANIAL NERVE

Common causes include diabetes, infarction, and trauma

If third nerve palsy is acute, MRI or conventional arteriography is required to exclude an aneurysm of the carotid or posterior communicating artery

Internal Disk Derangement of Temporomandibular Joint

Presenting Signs and Symptoms

Clicking or popping sound when opening the mouth (displacement with reduction)

Painful limitation of jaw movement (displacement without reduction)

Common Causes

Chronic spasm of the lateral pterygoid muscle
Trauma
Arthritic changes in articular surfaces

Approach to Diagnostic Imaging

▶ I. **Magnetic resonance imaging**
   ▶ Preferred modality for evaluating displacement of the disk and whether there is reduction during function (should be performed in the open- and closed-mouth positions using surface coils)

Note: Arthrography and CT are not as effective as MRI for imaging internal disk derangements of the temporomandibular joint.

BREAST

Edward A. Sickles

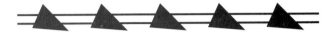

Breast Cancer

Presenting Signs and Symptoms

Asymptomatic (detected by screening with physical examination or mammography)

Variable clinical manifestations including mass, pain, breast enlargement, nipple discharge, nondescript thickening in the breast, lymphedema (peau d'orange), skin or nipple retraction, and evidence of matted or fixed axillary or supraclavicular lymph nodes

Risk Factors

MAJOR

Family history (first-degree relative, especially if premenopausal or bilateral)

Prior *in situ* or invasive breast cancer (risk of developing cancer in the contralateral breast after mastectomy is approximately 0.5–1% for every year of follow-up)

Prior biopsy showing atypical hyperplasia, especially in association with positive family history

MINOR

Early menarche

Late menopause

Late first pregnancy

Radiation exposure before the age of 30

Note: Possible but not definite minor risk factors include prolonged use of oral contraceptives before first pregnancy, postmenopausal estrogen replacement therapy, and high-fat diet.

Approach to Diagnostic Imaging

▶ **1. Mammography**
- ▶ Procedure of choice for detecting nonpalpable cancer because it demonstrates such early signs of malignancy as microcalcifications, small spiculated lesions, and subtle distortion of breast architecture
- ▶ Permits preoperative needle/wire localization of nonpalpable lesions that are suspicious for malignancy
- ▶ Allows assessment of the contralateral breast for clinically occult but mammographically suspicious abnormalities that should be biopsied concurrently

▶ **2. Ultrasound**
- ▶ If a mass detected on mammography may represent a cyst, ultrasound is indicated to make the critical distinction between a simple cyst (always benign and requiring no further work-up) and a complex or solid mass (may be malignant and requires further investigation)

 Caveat: Ultrasound *cannot* provide a definitive diagnosis of a solid or complex mass.

▶ **3. Fine-needle aspiration biopsy**
- ▶ Provides material for definitive cytologic examination

▶ **4. Core biopsy**
- ▶ Provides material for definitive histologic examination

Mammography Screening

American Cancer Society Guidelines

For women aged 40 to 49 years, a mammogram every *2 years* is recommended

For women older than age 50 years, *yearly* mammograms are recommended

---

Note: In recent screening studies including asymptomatic women, about 40% of cancers were detected by mammography but not physical examination. Conversely, about 10% of cancers were evident only on examination. Therefore, physical examination and mammography should be considered as *complementary* procedures.

 Caveats: Ultrasound, *not* used as a screening procedure, only makes the important distinction between simple cysts and solid masses.

Thermography, diaphanography, and transillumination should *never* be used for screening or diagnosis of breast disease.

Screening Outcomes

Note: Outcomes described are representative for 1,000 asymptomatic women undergoing bilateral screening mammography for the first time.

1. Will result in 70–100 (7–10%) being recalled for more studies (magnification or other special views; ultrasound)
2. In 15–20 (1.5–2%) biopsy will be required
3. In 5–7 (0.5–0.7%), cancer will be detected

Note: Of detected cancers, more than 30% will be minimal (ductal carcinoma *in situ* of any size; invasive cancer < 1 cm), and more than 70% will be node-negative.

Palpable Breast Mass

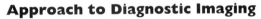

Approach to Diagnostic Imaging

▶ 1. **Mammography**
- ▶ Procedure of choice for determining whether the palpable mass is unequivocally benign (e.g., oil cyst, lipoma), thus avoiding biopsy
- ▶ If the palpable mass is suspicious for malignancy, the primary purpose of mammography is to assess the affected breast for multifocal disease and the contralateral breast for clinically occult but mammographically suspicious abnormalities that should be biopsied concurrently

Note: The palpable mass should always be indicated by placing a radiopaque marker over the site to assure that the palpable abnormality is included on available images and to determine whether it corresponds to any mammographic lesion that is visualized.

▶ 2. **Ultrasound**
- ▶ Indicated as a confirming procedure if mammography suggests that the palpable mass may represent a simple cyst. If rigid interpretive criteria are used, can be diagnostic of a simple (benign) cyst.
- ▶ Also indicated (as an alternative to fine-needle aspiration biopsy) to diagnose a simple cyst in a patient with a palpable mass and dense breasts who has a negative mammogram

 Caveat: Ultrasound *cannot* provide a definitive diagnosis of a solid or complex mass.

► 3. **Fine-needle aspiration biopsy**
  ► Provides material for definitive cytologic exam

 Caveat: In women *younger than age 30* who have a palpable mass, many radiologists prefer ultrasound as the initial imaging modality (because of the low incidence of breast cancer in this age group *and* the increased risk of breast cancer in women of this age who have received radiation). If the ultrasound is negative, a limited mammographic examination may then be performed to search for suspicious microcalcifications suggesting malignancy (that cannot be detected by ultrasound).

REPRODUCTIVE
Hedvig Hricak

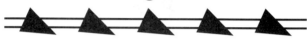

▶ SIGNS AND SYMPTOMS

Female
Abnormal Uterine
    Bleeding
Dysmenorrhea

Infertility
Missing Intrauterine
    Device (IUD)

Male
Scrotal Pain (Acute)

Undescended Testis
    (Cryptorchidism)

▶ DISORDERS

Female
Mass
    Cancer of the Cervix
    Cancer of the
        Endometrium
    Cancer of the Ovary
    Endometriosis

    Leiomyoma (Fibroid)
       of the Uterus
    Pelvic Mass
Other
    Adenomyosis
    Pelvic Inflammatory
       Disease (Salpingitis)

Male
Benign Prostatic
    Hyperplasia (BPH)

Cancer of the Prostate
Testicular Malignancy

Abnormal Uterine Bleeding

Presenting Signs and Symptoms

Excessive menstrual duration (menorrhagia)
Excessive menstrual amount (hypermenorrhea)
Nonmenstrual or intermenstrual bleeding (metrorrhagia)
Postmenopausal bleeding

Common Causes

Dysfunctional bleeding (75%) due to a functional abnormality of the hypothalamic-pituitary-ovarian axis)
Complication of pregnancy
Endometriosis
Vaginal lesion
Malignant neoplasm
Adenomyosis
Leiomyoma
Functional ovarian cysts
Contraceptives
Hematologic disorder with abnormal clotting

Approach to Diagnostic Imaging

► I. **Ultrasound**
   ► Preferred initial imaging procedure for detecting abnormalities of the female genital tract

---

Note: See individual sections for recommended work-up of specific disorders.

Dysmenorrhea

Presenting Sign and Symptom

Cyclic pain associated with menses during ovulatory cycles

Common Causes

Primary (no demonstrable lesion affecting the reproductive structures)

Secondary

Endometriosis

Chronic pelvic inflammatory disease

Cervical stenosis, infection, or neoplasm

Approach to Diagnostic Imaging

▶ I. Ultrasound
  ▶ Imaging procedure of choice for detecting or excluding lesions of the female genital tract

Infertility

Common Causes

MALE FACTORS (40%)
Deficient spermatogenesis
Varicocele
Cryptorchidism
Retrograde ejaculation into the bladder

FEMALE FACTORS (60%)
Ovulatory dysfunction (20%)
Tubal dysfunction (30%)
Cervical mucus dysfunction (5%)
Other (5%)

Approach to Diagnostic Imaging

▶ 1. **Hysterosalpingography**
- ▶ Preferred imaging study to demonstrate obstruction of the fallopian tubes (usually secondary to scarring from pelvic inflammatory disease); synechial adhesions; filling defects within the uterine cavity; and congenital anomalies

▶ 2. **Ultrasound or magnetic resonance imaging**
- ▶ Indicated if the hysterosalpingogram is normal in order to detect congenital anomalies of the female genital tract that are seen in up to 10% of women evaluated for infertility or repeated abortion

Missing Intrauterine Device (IUD)

Presenting Sign and Symptom

Patient unable to feel the attached string (and did not notice that the device was expelled)

Approach to Diagnostic Imaging

▶ 1. **Ultrasound**
   - ▶ Preferred screening technique if an intrauterine position of the device cannot be confirmed by pelvic examination, uterine sound, or biopsy instrument

▶ 2. **Lateral pelvic radiograph**
   - ▶ If the position of the IUD cannot be unequivocally determined by ultrasound, a single lateral view with contrast material in the uterine cavity can demonstrate whether an opaque IUD lies within or outside the uterus

---

Note: A plain frontal view is *not* sufficient because it can misdiagnose an extrauterine IUD located in the cul-de-sac.

Scrotal Pain (Acute)

Common Causes

Testicular torsion (usually occurs in patients younger than age 20; characterized by more acute onset)

Acute epididymo-orchitis (most common after age 20; more gradual onset, often with pyuria)

Vasculitis (e.g., Henoch-Schönlein purpura in children; polyarteritis nodosa in adults)

Trauma

Strangulated, incarcerated hernia

Approach to Diagnostic Imaging

▶ 1. **Ultrasound with color Doppler**
  - ▶ Demonstrates decreased or absent flow on the symptomatic side in torsion, compared with a diffuse increase in blood flow on the affected side in epididymo-orchitis

▶ 2. **Radionuclide flow study**
  - ▶ Demonstrates torsion as a rounded cold area surrounded by a rim of increased radionuclide activity reflecting hyperemia (doughnut sign), compared with generalized increase in vascular flow to the affected side in epididymo-orchitis

 Caveat: The choice of imaging technique is made on an individualized basis. The general preference is to use ultrasound in adults and radionuclide studies in children.

Undescended Testis (Cryptorchidism)

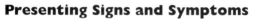

Presenting Signs and Symptoms

Incomplete or improper prenatal descent of one or both testes (occurs in about 3% of newborns; most spontaneously descend, so that by age 1 the incidence is only 1%)

Long-Term Complications (Requiring Orchiopexy)

Infertility due to progressive failure of spermatogenesis

Increased risk of a malignant testicular neoplasm developing (in both the undescended and in the contralateral, normally descended testis)

Approach to Diagnostic Imaging

Note: The use of diagnostic imaging for nonpalpable undescended testes is highly controversial, with some surgeons preferring to go directly to laparoscopy or operative exploration.

▶ I. Ultrasound
  ▶ Sensitive for demonstrating the often-atrophic undescended testis if it is located beyond the internal inguinal ring (inguinal canal and spermatic cord)

Note: Identification of the mediastinum testis is important to distinguish an undescended testis from an enlarged lymph node in the area of the cord.

 Caveat: Ultrasound is of *no* value if the testis is located in the pelvis or abdomen.

▶ **2. Computed tomography**

  ▶ Most valuable for detecting the undescended abdominal testis; may also be of use in the postpubertal male or if neoplastic degeneration is suspected

 Caveat: CT involves radiation (a consideration in this generally younger age group) and cannot detect an undescended testis smaller than 1 cm.

▶ **3. Magnetic resonance imaging**

  ▶ Preferred approach for detecting undescended testes located at or beyond the internal ring of the inguinal canal, and for demonstrating all complications (especially inflammatory or neoplastic)

Cancer of the Cervix

Presenting Signs and Symptoms

Usually detected by screening Papanicolaou (Pap) test
Vaginal discharge and bleeding

Risk Factors

History of early, frequent coitus and multiple partners
Possible relationship to venereal transmission of human
   papilloma virus (HPV)

Staging

▶ 1. **Magnetic resonance imaging**
  - ▶ Preferred study for demonstrating the tumor, measuring its size, and showing direct tumor extension to the vagina, paracervical, and parametrial tissues, bladder, and rectum
  - ▶ MRI is superior to CT, which even with contrast enhancement cannot consistently differentiate tumor from adjacent normal tissue

▶ 2. **Computed tomography**
  - ▶ Valuable in advanced disease and in the search for lymph node metastases

 Caveat: Cervical cancer frequently metastasizes to pelvic, inguinal, and retroperitoneal lymph nodes but may not enlarge them. However, both MRI and CT use lymph node enlargement as primary criterion for detecting metastatic involvement.

▶ 3. **Endovaginal ultrasound**
  ▶ Can assess tumor size (but is inferior to MRI)

 Caveat: There is *no* indication for the routine use of excretory urography or barium enema examination (the diagnostic mainstays before cross-sectional imaging).

Cancer of the Endometrium

Presenting Signs and Symptoms

Inappropriate uterine bleeding (postmenopausal or recurrent metrorrhagia in a premenopausal woman)
Mucoid or watery discharge

Predisposing Factors

Estrogen-producing ovarian tumor
Delayed menopause
Abnormal menstrual history or infertility

Possible Implicated Factors

Obesity
Hypertension
Diabetes mellitus
Breast cancer
Absence of ovulation
Family history of breast or ovarian cancer

Approach to Diagnostic Imaging

▶ I. **Ultrasound (endovaginal approach preferred)**
    ▶ Used by some physicians to measure endometrial
thickness in postmenopausal women to select
patients suspected of having endometrial carcinoma for dilation and curettage (endometrial
stripe greater than 5 mm is an indication for endometrial biopsy)

Staging

▶ 1. **Magnetic resonance imaging**
  ▶ Procedure of choice to demonstrate the depth of myometrial invasion as well as extension into the cervix, broad ligaments, parametrium and ovaries, and lymphatic spread to pelvic and retroperitoneal lymph nodes

Note: MRI staging is superior to clinical evaluation and CT.

▶ 2. **Computed tomography**
  ▶ Indicated only in advanced cases to search for adjacent organ and pelvic side wall invasion or lymph node metastases

Note: Endovaginal ultrasound has been advocated for the assessment of myometrial invasion. However, this method has not been widely accepted because it is subjective and markedly operator dependent.

Cancer of the Ovary

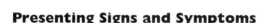

Presenting Signs and Symptoms

Asymptomatic (until very large)
Vague lower abdominal discomfort
Mild digestive complaints
Inappropriate vaginal bleeding
Late findings include abdominal swelling due to ascites and a lobulated, fixed solid mass associated with nodular implants in the cul-de-sac

Approach to Diagnostic Imaging

▶ I. **Ultrasound**
  ▶ Preferred screening procedure to demonstrate the usually large lesion that varies in appearance from a multilocular cyst with thin septations to a complex mass with prominent solid elements

---

Note: The value of endovaginal ultrasound using color flow Doppler to detect neovascularity in the ovary in the hope of earlier detection of ovarian cancer is controversial.

 Caveat: Although the risk of malignancy increases with the amount of solid tissue within the mass, in the absence of metastatic disease neither ultrasound nor any other imaging method can unequivocally differentiate benign from malignant ovarian masses.

▶ **2. Magnetic resonance imaging or computed tomography**
  ▸ Indicated when the ultrasound findings are inconclusive in determining whether a lesion is benign or malignant

Staging

▶ **I. Computed tomography**
  ▸ Preferred study for demonstrating direct extension of tumor to adjacent structures, peritoneal and omental spread, lymphatic metastases to pelvic and retroperitoneal nodes, malignant ascites, and late hematogenous spread to the liver and lung
  ▸ Currently considered superior to MRI because with the latter there has been difficulty in differentiating tumor from bowel, longer examination time, and higher cost

 Caveat: Ovarian carcinoma spreads primarily by peritoneal seeding, with small tumor nodules implanting on the peritoneum, mesentery, and omentum. Unfortunately, no imaging method is effective in detecting implants smaller than 2 to 3 cm in the absence of ascites, or smaller than 0.5 to 1.0 cm if ascites is present.

Note: MRI is indicated only if there is a contraindication to the use of iodinated contrast material (e.g., renal failure or allergy) or if the CT findings are inconclusive.

Endometriosis

Presenting Signs and Symptoms

Pelvic pain associated with menses (dysmenorrhea)
Dyspareunia
Pelvic mass
Effect of implants on other organs (lesions involving large bowel or bladder may cause pain with defecation, abdominal bloating, rectal bleeding with menses, or hematuria and suprapubic pain during urination)

Common Causes

Unknown mechanism for presence of endometrial tissue at ectopic sites outside the uterine cavity (retrograde flow of menstrual bleeding is a hypothesis)

Predisposing Factors

Family history
Delay in childbearing
Müllerian duct anomalies
Oriental race

Approach to Diagnostic Imaging

 Caveat: Ectopic implants of endometrial tissue generally are too small to be visualized by any imaging method, and laparoscopy is essential for their detection and for staging of endometriosis.

▶ I. **Ultrasound**
 ▶ May demonstrate cystic mass(es) filled with old blood (endometrioma)

Note: Although ultrasound can identify the presence of an adnexal lesion, it may be unable to differentiate definitively an endometrioma from other adnexal masses.

▶ 2. **Magnetic resonance imaging**
  ▶ Most sensitive modality for diagnosing endometriosis and for differentiating an endometrioma from other adnexal masses

Notes: MRI cannot reliably visualize adhesions or intraperitoneal implants.

Other imaging modalities (barium enema, excretory urography, CT) may demonstrate the extent of disease (secondary involvement of other organs) and response to therapy but are not sufficiently specific to provide a precise diagnosis.

Leiomyoma (Fibroid) of the Uterus

Presenting Signs and Symptoms

Note: Signs and symptoms depend on the location and size of the lesion.

Asymptomatic (detected incidentally on routine pelvic examination or imaging study performed for other reason)

Inappropriate vaginal bleeding

Pressure symptoms caused by increasing size of the uterus

Acute abdomen (when torsed or undergoing "red" degeneration)

Approach to Diagnostic Imaging

▶ 1. **Ultrasound**
   ▸ Preferred imaging technique for diagnosing this benign uterine tumor (endovaginal studies are helpful for submucosal leiomyomas)

    Caveat: There is no longer any indication for the use of hysterosalpingography to diagnose submucosal leiomyomas.

▶ 2. **Magnetic resonance imaging**
   ▸ Indicated if the ultrasound examination is negative or inconclusive in differentiating between uterine and adnexal masses; if the mass is unusually large; to search for submucosal leiomyomas; in an infertility work-up; and in distinguishing between leiomyoma and adenomyosis

Note: MRI is more sensitive than either ultrasound or hysterosalpingography.

 Caveat: Neither ultrasound nor **MRI** can reliably differentiate benign leiomyoma from the rare malignant leiomyosarcoma.

Note: Although not indicated for imaging of clinically suspected leiomyoma, plain abdominal radiographs may fortuitously detect the lesion by demonstrating the virtually pathognomonic "popcorn" pattern of pelvic calcification.

Pelvic Mass

Presenting Sign and Symptom

Palpable or clinically suspected mass

Approach to Diagnostic Imaging

▶ 1. **Ultrasound**
  - ▸ Preferred imaging procedure for evaluating the patient with a pelvic mass
  - ▸ Can confirm the presence of a mass, establish its organ of origin, and demonstrate its internal consistency (cystic, complex, or solid)

 Caveat: Ultrasound is less accurate than CT or MRI for demonstrating tumor extension of a malignant neoplasm or lymph node metastases.

▶ 2. **Computed tomography or magnetic resonance imaging**
  - ▸ Preferred imaging methods for further evaluating pelvic tumors and for staging pelvic masses suspected of being malignant
  - ▸ Superior to ultrasound for demonstrating tumor spread to adjacent and distant structures

Note: The role of excretory urography has been limited to assessing those patients with pelvic masses who also have hematuria. If the patient presents with renal failure, the presence of hydronephrosis can be established by ultrasound. If there is suspicion of a malignant lesion, contrast CT can adequately evaluate renal function and the path of the ureters.

 Caveat: There is *no* indication for plain abdominal radiographs (too insensitive and nonspecific).

Adenomyosis

Presenting Signs and Symptoms

Menorrhagia and intermenstrual bleeding
Globular enlargement of the uterus
Nonspecific pelvic pain and bladder and rectal pressure

Common Cause

Benign invasion of endometrium (basalis layer) into the myometrium

Approach to Diagnostic Imaging

▶ 1. **Ultrasound**
- ▶ Endovaginal sonography is the recommended initial imaging procedure to demonstrate the heterogeneous texture of an enlarged uterus

 Caveat: On ultrasound, many patients with a leiomyomatous uterus have a similar pattern of diffusely abnormal uterine texture without evidence of discrete leiomyomas. When surgery is planned, distinguishing between leiomyoma and adenomyosis is crucial in patients who wish to preserve the uterus. Adenomyosis requires hysterectomy for definitive therapy, whereas leiomyomas can be treated by selective myomectomy with preservation of the uterus.

▶ 2. **Magnetic resonance imaging**
- ▶ Highly sensitive for detecting adenomyosis and accurate in making the critical distinction from leiomyoma

---

Note: CT is *not* applicable in this clinical situation.

Pelvic Inflammatory Disease (Salpingitis)

Presenting Signs and Symptoms

ACUTE

Lower abdominal pain, fever, and purulent vaginal discharge that usually begins shortly after menses

CHRONIC

Chronic pain, menstrual irregularities, and infertility (due to mucosal destruction and tubal obstruction)

Common Sources of Infection

Sexual intercourse, childbirth (puerperal fever), abortion

Note: Patients with IUDs are particularly susceptible.

Approach to Diagnostic Imaging

Note: In uncomplicated cases that respond well to antibiotic therapy, there is *no* need for imaging studies.

▶ 1. **Ultrasound**
   ▶ To demonstrate pyosalpinx or tubo-ovarian abscess complicating pelvic inflammatory disease (and to assess their response to therapy)

▶ 2. **Computed tomography**
   ▶ May be performed after ultrasound to visualize the full extent of disease in severe cases
   ▶ Indicated if clinical symptoms mimic appendicitis

Note: MRI is used only if CT is indicated and the patient is allergic to iodinated contrast material.

Benign Prostatic Hyperplasia (BPH)

Presenting Signs and Symptoms

Varying degrees of bladder outlet obstruction (progressive urinary frequency, urgency, and nocturia due to incomplete emptying and refilling of the bladder)

Decreased size and force of the urinary stream (associated with hesitancy and intermittency)

May have terminal dribbling, almost continuous overflow incontinence, or complete urinary retention

Common Causes

Unknown (may involve hormonal imbalance associated with aging)

Approach to Diagnostic Imaging

Note: BPH is a *clinical* diagnosis, indicating imaging when volume of gland is a determinant in deciding the surgical approach, to follow changes in size of the gland during medical therapy, and if there is a need to assess the degree of urinary obstruction. The size of the gland does *not* correlate with the symptoms.

▶ I. **Ultrasound**
  ▶ *Transrectal* sonography demonstrates enlargement and heterogeneity of the gland (specifically the transitional zone) and often shows a circumferential pseudocapsule. Discrete nodules may be visualized, as well as nodular thickening of the bladder wall.
  ▶ *Transabdominal* sonography is used to measure the residual urine volume and to evaluate the kidney for the presence of hydronephrosis

► **2. Excretory urography**
  ► Demonstrates a filling defect at the base of the bladder associated with upward displacement of the terminal portions of the ureters (fishhooking)
  ► Can assess the degree of urinary obstruction

Cancer of the Prostate

Presenting Signs and Symptoms

Asymptomatic

May be symptoms of bladder outlet obstruction, ureteral obstruction, hematuria, and pyuria (indistinguishable from benign prostatic hyperplasia)

Elevated prostate-specific antigen (PSA)

Localized bone pain (from common skeletal metastases)

Elevated serum acid phosphatase (indicates local extension or metastases)

Common Causes

Probably hormone related

Approach to Diagnostic Imaging

▶ I. **Transrectal ultrasound**

- ▶ Preferred imaging technique once prostatic carcinoma has been suspected by digital rectal examination or elevated prostate specific antigen

- ▶ Suspicious signs of malignancy include a hypoechoic nodule (especially in the peripheral zone), mass effect on surrounding tissues, and asymmetric enlargement of the gland with deformation of its contour. However, none of these findings are specific for malignancy

- ▶ Gland volume measurements from imaging are necessary to calculate the PSA density (gland volume/PSA)

- ▶ Excellent for guiding needle biopsy

 Caveats: Up to 25% of prostate cancers are isoechoic and indistinguishable from normal parenchyma. In addition, it is difficult for any imaging modality to detect cancer in the midst of benign prostatic hyperplasia.

There is *no* indication for excretory urography in the evaluation of the patient with suspected prostate cancer.

There also is *no* indication for **MRI in the** *pre*-biopsy investigation for prostate cancer. MRI can detect many tumors, but there is an overlap in the MRI appearance of malignant and benign prostate nodules and a precise diagnosis requires biopsy and histologic examination.

Staging

▶ 1. **Magnetic resonance imaging**
   ▸ The use of phased-array coils, endorectal coils, or a combination represents the state-of-the-art and most effective imaging technique for assessing local and regional spread (extracapsular extension, seminal vesicle invasion) and metastatic involvement of lymph nodes

▶ 2. **Computed tomography**
   ▸ Although once considered the gold standard for staging of prostate cancer, this modality is no longer used routinely. CT staging is recommended only if the presence of lymph node metastases is suggested on clinical grounds (markedly abnormal digital rectal examination and PSA)

▶ 3. **Radionuclide bone scan**
   ▸ The single best modality for detecting skeletal metastases (high frequency with prostatic cancer)

 Caveat: Radionuclide bone scans are no longer recommended routinely. They should be ordered only if the **PSA** exceeds 10 or if there are skeletal symptoms.

Testicular Malignancy

Presenting Signs and Symptoms

Scrotal mass (progressively increasing in size)

Generally painless (may be exquisite pain if hemorrhage into a rapidly expanding tumor)

Often attributed to minor trauma (indicating the time when the mass was first discovered)

Approach to Diagnostic Imaging

▶ 1. **Ultrasound**

> ▶ Primary imaging adjunct to physical examination that localizes the mass to the testis and characterizes its internal composition

▶ 2. **Magnetic resonance imaging**

> ▶ Problem-solving modality performed if ultrasound is equivocal; if there is a discrepancy between the physical examination and the ultrasound study; if bilateral disease is likely (e.g., lymphoma, leukemia); or as follow-up of the patient with a unilateral testis and an equivocal ultrasound study

Staging

▶ 1. **Computed tomography (abdomen and pelvis)**

> ▶ Most effective staging procedure for demonstrating the presence and extent of extratesticular spread of tumor (most commonly through the lymphatic system along the gonadal vessels following the testicular veins to renal hilar nodes on the left or the aortocaval chain on the right or along the external iliac chain)

Note: Thin-section CT of the lungs is also recommended for early detection of the frequent pulmonary metastases.

▶**2. Magnetic resonance imaging**
  ▶ Comparable to CT for detecting retroperitoneal lymphadenopathy. Possible advantages of MRI include the ability to distinguish lymph nodes from blood vessels without the use of intravenous contrast material
  ▶ Recommended in patients with elevated creatinine, allergy to iodinated contrast material, or retroperitoneal surgical clips (which would degrade the CT image)

OBSTETRICS

Peter W. Callen

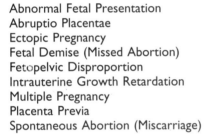

Abnormal Fetal Presentation

Approach to Diagnostic Imaging

▶ I. **Ultrasound**
   ▶ Preferred study for detecting breech presentation

Note: There is *no* indication for plain abdominal radiographs to establish the position of the fetal skull.

Abruptio Placentae

Presenting Signs and Symptoms

Vary depending on the degree of placental separation and the extent of blood loss

Third-trimester bleeding (retroplacental hemorrhage that may pass through the cervix and produce vaginal bleeding or be retained behind the placenta)

Severe bleeding may lead to fetal cardiac distress or death and maternal shock

Complications include disseminated intravascular coagulation, acute renal failure, and uteroplacental apoplexy

Risk Factors

Maternal hypertension
Smoking
Cocaine abuse
Autoimmune disorders
Previous history of abruptio placentae

Approach to Diagnostic Imaging

▶ I. **Ultrasound**
  ▸ Major value is to exclude a placenta previa as the cause of vaginal bleeding
  ▸ May often miss the diagnosis of abruptio placentae due to (1) complete egress of retroplacental blood or (2) isoechogenicity of blood compared to the placenta
  ▸ *Retro*placental clot may sometimes be recognized sonographically. An abnormally thickened placenta in the absence of hydrops fetalis should raise the suspicion of *intra*placental extension of blood

Ectopic Pregnancy

Presenting Signs and Symptoms

Cramping pelvic pain
Spotting (occasionally rapid bleeding leading to shock)
Enlarged uterus but smaller than expected for dates
May be tender mass in one adnexa
Lower-than-expected HCG level

Predisposing Factors

Pelvic inflammatory disease
Tubal surgery
Endometriosis
Ovulation induction
Previous ectopic pregnancy
Exposure to diethylstilbestrol (DES)

Approach to Diagnostic Imaging

▶ 1. **Ultrasound**
- ▶ Procedure of choice for demonstrating the extra-uterine gestational sac, empty uterus, and secondary signs of ectopic pregnancy
- ▶ A normal sonogram still carries as much as a 20% risk of an ectopic pregnancy (even if endovaginal sonography is used)

Note: When an intrauterine pregnancy is demonstrated by ultrasound, the risk of a coexisting ectopic pregnancy is extremely low (about 1 in 17,000–30,000). Nevertheless, concurrent intrauterine and ectopic pregnancies do occur, especially in women taking ovulation-inducing drugs.

Fetal Demise
(Missed Abortion)

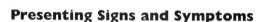

Presenting Signs and Symptoms

Failure of the uterus to grow

Absence of fetal heart tone (either if not heard at an appropriate time or if a previously present fetal heart sound can no longer be heard)

Decreasing HCG levels

Approach to Diagnostic Imaging

▶ I. **Ultrasound**

    ▶ Confirms the diagnosis by indicating the absence of fetal cardiac activity at a time when it should have been detectable

---

Note: Using endovaginal techniques, absence of cardiac activity in embryos larger than 5 mm is considered diagnostic of fetal demise. Embryos smaller than 5 mm without cardiac activity should be rescanned in a few days to confirm demise.

Fetopelvic Disproportion

Presenting Sign and Symptom

Failure of proper descent of the fetal head into the pelvis

Common Causes

Malpositioned fetal head (e.g., breech presentation, hyperextended fetal head)

Inadequate maternal pelvis

Approach to Diagnostic Imaging

▶ 1. **Computed tomography**
  ▶ Sagittal and coronal digital radiographs of the pelvis combined with a single-slice axial CT image is the procedure of choice for efficient assessment of pelvic and fetal measurements

---

Note: This technique has higher accuracy and produces far less radiation exposure to both the fetus and the mother than conventional pelvimetry.

Intrauterine Growth Retardation (IUGR)

Presenting Sign and Symptom

Estimated fetal weight below the 10th percentile for gestational age

Common Causes

Short parents

Fetal chromosomal abnormalities

Intrauterine infection (cytomegalovirus, rubella, toxoplasmosis)

Maternal disease (hypertension, preeclampsia, diabetes mellitus, renal disease, malnutrition)

Smoking, alcohol, drug abuse

Approach to Diagnostic Imaging

▶ I. **Ultrasound**

- ▶ Preferred imaging study to initially estimate the gestational age of the fetus and assess whether fetal growth is proceeding normally
- ▶ Can distinguish *symmetric* IUGR (which may be related to chromosome abnormalities or intrauterine infection), in which the head, abdomen, and femur measurements are all proportionally small from *asymmetric* IUGR (related to maternal disorders), in which the fetal abdomen is disproportionally small relative to the head and femur
- ▶ Demonstrates the oligohydramnios associated with severe IUGR

Multiple Pregnancy

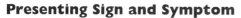

Presenting Sign and Symptom

Large uterine size for dates

Approach to Diagnostic Imaging

▶ 1. **Ultrasound**
  - ▶ Demonstrates the presence of multiple embryos or fetuses
  - ▶ Permits characterization of multiple pregnancies according to the number of amniotic sacs and whether or not the fetuses share a single placenta

---

Note: The relative risk of twin morbidity (prematurity, polyhydramnios, increased incidence of congenital anomalies, discordant growth, cord accidents) is substantially higher if the fetuses share a placenta (monochorionic) and a single amniotic cavity (monoamniotic).

Placenta Previa

Presenting Signs and Symptoms

Painless third-trimester vaginal bleeding (may become massive, bright red bleeding)

> **Note:** May be indistinguishable from abruptio placentae.

Risk Factors

Previous cesarean section

Uterine abnormality inhibiting normal implantation (fibroid)

Multiple previous pregnancies

Previous placenta previa

Approach to Diagnostic Imaging

 Caveat: It is critical to make the distinction between placenta previa and abruptio placentae. Until the diagnosis of abruptio placentae has been definitely established, vaginal examination is *contraindicated* due to the risk that it might precipitate greater hemorrhage in the patient with placenta previa.

▶ I. **Ultrasound**
  ▶ Procedure of choice to demonstrate that part or all of the placenta covers the internal cervical os in a woman in the *third* trimester

> **Note:** Transperineal (translabial) ultrasound may greatly enhance visualization of the cervix, lower uterine segment, and placental edge.

Spontaneous Abortion (Miscarriage)

Presenting Signs and Symptoms

Delivery or loss of the products of conception before the 20th week of pregnancy

Common Causes

Fetal chromosomal abnormality

Maternal causes

Cervical abnormality (incompetent, amputated, or lacerated)

Uterine abnormality (leiomyoma, congenital anomaly)

Impaired corpus luteum function

Hypothyroidism

Diabetes mellitus

Chronic renal disease

Infection (especially viruses such as cytomegalovirus, rubella, and herpes)

Approach to Diagnostic Imaging

▶ I. **Ultrasound**

 ▶ Procedure of choice to demonstrate a gestational sac without an embryo or yolk sac or to show a retained nonviable pregnancy

 ▶ Can demonstrate an underlying structural abnormality involving the uterus

Appendix I

Digital Radiography (Computed Radiography)

There is currently an increasing trend toward the use of Picture Archiving and Communications Systems (PACS), which utilize digital images rather than traditional x-ray films. Although this approach is ideally suited to the newer digital imaging modalities (ultrasound, CT, MRI, and radionuclide studies), conventional radiography presents a significant obstacle. Whether obtained in the main radiology department of a hospital, the operating suite, or as portable examinations on extremely ill patients, plain radiographs of the chest, abdomen, and skeletal structures are generally obtained in an analog mode. The following systems are the main approaches now being used to digitize these analog images and make them PACS-compatible.

DIGITAL CONVERSION OF CONVENTIONAL RADIOGRAPHIC IMAGES (AFTER EXPOSURE AND DEVELOPMENT). Among the many disadvantages of this approach are the high cost (requires twice the number of films for each examination) and the relatively long time required for digital conversion (only a small number of films can be handled). Automatic loading is expensive and complicated because of the many different sizes of films. Manual loading presents even more problems. Because of these drawbacks, digital conversion of conventional radiographic images is not generally used.

PHOTO-STIMULABLE PHOSPHOR RADIOGRAPHY ("FUJI APPROACH"). First introduced in 1981, this technique is based on the storing of two-dimensional information created by x-rays on a photo-stimulable plate the same size as the object. After the plate is illuminated with laser beams, the information it contains is released as photo-stimulated luminescence that is converted into an analog electronic read-out by a photo-multiplier. The analog signal obtained is then converted into a digital image. The photo-stimulable plate is reusable, since the image is erased once the laser light releases the stored electrons.

The photo-stimulable phosphor method has been licensed by Fuji to many companies and is currently in wide use. The major disadvantage, however, is the great expense of the photo-stimulable plates, as well as the rest of the system.

IMAGE INTENSIFICATION. By using an image intensifier of sufficient size to capture the image of the subject, the luminescent image created by photo-multiplication can then be digitized. The disadvantage of this approach is the difficulty encountered in manufacturing the required 17″ × 17″ high-resolution, artifact-free, uniform-surface image intensifiers at an acceptable cost.

SPECIAL APPROACHES. CT scanners can directly create digital radiographs. This technique is primarily used for pelvimetry, in which sagittal and coronal scout digital radiographs of the pelvis are obtained along with a single-plane transverse image. However, this method of obtaining digital images is far too costly for general use. In addition, it would not provide adequate detail, since the CT matrix is too coarse to produce high-resolution radiographs.

Ultrasound

Ultrasound is the most popular and widely acceptable cross-sectional imaging technique. It combines relatively low cost with wide distribution, immediate accessibility, high spatial resolution, and the ability to image in any plane. In this noninvasive modality, high-frequency sound waves produced by electrical stimulation of a specialized crystal are passed through the body (reduced in intensity) in relation to the acoustic properties of the tissues through which they travel. The crystal is mounted in a transducer, which also acts as a receiver to record echoes that are reflected back from the body whenever the sound wave strikes an interface between two tissues that have different acoustic impedance. A water-tissue interface produces strong reflections (echoes), whereas a solid-tissue mass that contains only small differences in composition causes weak reflections. The display of the ultrasound image on a television monitor shows both the intensity level of the echoes and the position in the body from which they arose. Ultrasound images may be displayed as static gray-scale images or as multiple images that permit movement to be viewed in "real-time." In general, fluid-filled structures have intense echoes at their borders, no internal echoes, and good through transmission of the sound waves. Solid structures produce internal echoes of variable intensity.

The last technology in ultrasound is the color flow duplex system, in which conventional real-time imaging is combined with Doppler imaging (to produce quantitative data) as well as color to depict motion and the direction and velocity of blood flow. The color and intensity represent the direction of flow and the magnitude of the velocity, respectively.

The major advantage of ultrasound is its safety. To date, there is no evidence of adverse effects on human tissues at the intensity level currently used for diagnostic procedures. Therefore, ultrasound is the modality of choice for the examination of children and pregnant women, in whom there is potential danger from the radiation exposure of most other imaging studies. It is by far the best technique for evaluating fetal age, congenital anomalies, and complications of pregnancy. The major limitation of ultrasound is the presence of acoustic barriers, such as air, bone, and barium. For example, air reflects essentially all of the ultrasound beam, so that structures beneath it cannot be imaged. This is a special problem in a patient with adynamic ileus and is the major factor precluding the ultrasound examination of the thorax. For a sonographic study of the pelvis, the patient is usually given large amounts of fluid to fill the bladder, thus displacing the air-filled bowel from the region of interest.

In the postoperative patient, ultrasound may be difficult to perform because of overlying dressings, retention sutures, drains, and open wounds that may prevent the transducer from coming into direct contact with the skin.

Ultrasound is also highly operator-dependent. Extensive technologist training is necessary to produce high-quality images suitable for interpretation.

Computed Tomography (CT)

In this technique, cross-sectional tomographic images are obtained by first scanning a "slice" of tissue from multiple angles with a narrow x-ray beam, then calculating a relative linear attenuation coefficient (amount of radiation absorbed in tissue for the various tissue elements in the section), and finally displaying the computed reconstruction of hundreds of thousands of bits of data as a gray-scale image on a television monitor.

The CT number reflects the attenuation of a specific tissue relative to that of water, which is arbitrarily given a CT number of 0. The highest CT number is that of bone; the lowest is of air. Fat has a CT number of less than 0, whereas soft tissues have CT numbers greater than 0.

The major advantages of CT (especially when enhanced with oral and intravenous iodinated contrast material) over conventional and digital radiography are its superb contrast resolution, speed, and the ability to display exquisite anatomic detail in tomographic form.

The newest technology in CT is spiral scanning. In this technique, continual CT scanning is performed as the patient is moved through the gantry (unlike the multiple single scans in conventional CT). This permits much faster scanning with substantial reduction of artifacts due to respiratory motion. Spiral scanning provides data that can be reformatted in coronal and sagittal planes and offers the potential of demonstrating vascular lesions without the need for arteriography.

Because of its many advantages, CT is now competing with ultrasound as the screening modality of choice in the developed world. The only real disadvantages of CT are its relatively high cost and the use of ionizing radiation.

Magnetic Resonance Imaging (MRI)

This rapidly developing imaging technique basically consists of inducing transitions between energy states by causing certain hydrogen atoms within a powerful static magnetic field to absorb and transfer energy when impacted by a radio pulse of a specific frequency. Various measures of the time required for the material to return to a baseline energy state (relaxation time) can be translated by a complex computer program to a visual image on a television monitor. The parameters of the MR image are set by selection of a pulse sequence. Most magnets used for MRI are superconducting (cryogenic). However, to reduce cost some equipment uses permanent or resistive magnets.

Although the signal intensity of various substances on MR scans is complex and depends on multiple factors, some generalizations can be made. On T1-weighted images, substances causing high signal intensity (bright) include fat, subacute hemorrhage, highly proteinaceous material (e.g., mucus), and slow-flowing blood. Water, as in cerebrospinal fluid or simple cysts, has a relatively low signal intensity and appears dark. Soft tissue has an intermediate level of signal. On T2-weighted images, water has a high signal intensity (bright), whereas muscle and other soft tissues (including fat) tend to have a low signal intensity and appear dark. Bone, calcium, and air appear very dark on all imaging sequences.

MRI has many of the advantages offered by other imaging modalities, without the associated disadvantages. Like ultrasound, MRI does not use ionizing radiation and is capable of directly imaging in multiple planes. Unlike ultrasound, MRI depends less on the operator's skill and can penetrate bone and air without a significant decrease in intensity so that the underlying tissue can be clearly imaged. Major advantages of MRI over CT are the far higher soft-tissue contrast resolution, the ability to directly image in any plane, the capacity to depict patent blood vessels as signal voids without the need for iodinated contrast material, and the use of innumerable different sequences to improve soft-tissue contrast and reduce artifacts.

Although MRI has improved the sensitivity of detecting abnormal tissue, it has had much less effect on specificity. In the head, for example, infarction, edema, tumor, infection, and demyelinating disease all produce identical high signal intensity on T2-weighted images. Other disadvantages of MRI include its high cost; a slower scanning time, leading to image degradation resulting from patient motion, and difficulty in studying the lung, gastrointestinal tract, and mesentery; the possibility of patient claustrophobia; and the contraindication to imaging patients with pacemakers (may prevent proper operation) or intracranial ferromagnetic aneurysm clips (may slip and result in hemorrhage). New approaches to motion suppression are constantly being developed. Ultrafast techniques for MRI scanning are now available that effectively trade speed for spatial resolution.

MR angiography is a new technique that provides high-quality images of the arterial and venous systems without the need for contrast material. Further technical refinements and clinical experience will expand the role of this modality and may allow MR angiography to eventually supplant contrast angiography in the diagnosis of vascular disease.

MRI has emerged as the imaging modality of choice for evaluating the central nervous system (brain and spinal cord), musculoskeletal system (including joints and spine), pelvis, retroperitoneum, mediastinum, and large vessels. It is equivalent to contrast-enhanced CT for studying focal liver disease, lymphadenopathy, and disorders of the spleen, pancreas, and kidneys.

In specific clinical situations (such as most disease processes involving the central nervous system), it is more cost-effective to perform MRI as the initial imaging procedure to achieve a precise diagnosis, rather than obtaining numerous other imaging studies and then having to order an MRI scan anyway.

Contrast Media

Contrast media are employed in medical imaging to increase contrast between various tissues, to depict the hollow viscera, to study blood vessels and the flow within them, to assess organ function, and to facilitate interventional procedures. Contrast media are widely used with all imaging modalities except ultrasound (though even in this area vascuar applications are now being developed and tested prior to FDA approval).

BARIUM SULFATE. This inert material is used as a suspension in water primarily to study the gastrointestinal tract. Suspending agents are employed to prevent sedimentation and flocculation. Double-contrast techniques using air (or methylcellulose in enteroclysis) provide superb depiction of mucosal surface detail.

WATER-SOLUBLE, IODINATED CONTRAST MEDIA. These chemicals can directly visualize the blood vessels (arteriography, venography) or opacify the urinary tract after being excreted by the kidneys. The use of newer, relatively expensive, low osmolar or nonionic contrast material can reduce the minor complications and the painful and unpleasant symptoms that may commonly follow the injection of hypertonic iodine-containing contrast media. It is unclear whether these newer substances also can reduce the mortality rate of 1 in 100,000 administrations associated with conventional hypertonic iodinated contrast material.

The American College of Radiology recommends the use of nonionic contrast media in patients with (1) history of adverse reaction to iodinated contrast material, (2) history of asthma or allergy, (3) known cardiac dysfunction, (4) generalized debilitation, or (5) whenever the radiologist believes that these contrast media are indicated.

Water-soluble contrast media are now most frequently used to increase contrast resolution in CT scanning. They can indicate whether an area of abnormality has increased or decreased vascularity compared with adjacent normal tissue. In the brain, contrast enhancement implies that there has been a break in the blood-brain barrier.

Water-soluble contrast material is used in routine radiography to demonstrate fistulas, sinuses, and perforations. As an enema, they are used when colonic perforation is suspected or in cases of severe constipation to soften hard stool.

MR CONTRAST AGENTS. At the present time, intravascular, extracellular chelates of gadolinium are used as tissue-enhancing agents to produce effects similar to those of iodinated contrast media in CT. They permit diagnoses that otherwise would require long T2-weighted images to be made on shorter T1-weighted sequences, thus reducing motion artifact. MR contrast agents are far safer than even the nonionic iodinated compounds used in conventional radiography and CT. Their major disadvantage is high cost, especially when added to the already steep price of MRI.

There is a substantial need for an orally administered MR contrast medium to outline the gastrointestinal tract. Currently, only one very costly agent containing bromine (no protons and thus no signal) has been FDA-approved for MRI.

Nuclear Medicine Instrumentation

SCINTILLATION CAMERA (ANGER CAMERA). This instrument consists of one, two, or three large, flat sodium iodide crystals up to 50 cm in diameter. Photons from the radioactive tracer produce luminescence in the crystal, which is then augmented many times by a large number of arrayed photomultiplier tubes. The two-dimensional location of the source of the signal, which is determined by computing the relative intensity of luminescence emitted by the multiple photo tubes, is displayed on an oscilloscope and then recorded on film.

SINGLE PHOTON EMISSION TOMOGRAPHY (SPECT). In this technique, the detector system rotates around the patient. The signal from the radioactive sources within the body is acquired from multiple projections and integrated using a computer algorithm somewhat similar to but more complicated than that used for CT.

POSITRON EMISSION TOMOGRAPHY (PET). Positron emitting materials such as C_{10}, C_{11}, or O_{15} have fewer neutrons than protons. They are produced in generators or cyclotrons by bombardment of atoms with protons or deuterons. Many are extremely short-lived. When a positron-emitting isotope is introduced into the body, it enters into annihilation reactions with electrons to produce a pair of gamma photons (each with an energy of 511 keV). These gamma photons radiate linearly in opposite directions at an angle of 180°. When they excite a circle of detectors, the signals are transferred into an image using an algorithm similar to that used in CT.

PET scanning is primarily employed to provide metabolic information. Its disadvantages are the relatively poor spatial resolution and the extremely high price of the examination.

Appendix II

With the ever-escalating cost of medicine, it is important to be constantly aware of the patient charges for different tests and procedures ordered. Knowing the price of these studies could lead to a reduction in unwarranted examinations and serve as an impetus to decreasing health care costs through a well-reasoned approach to diagnostic imaging.

Although less-expensive procedures sometimes yield approximately the same results as the more costly studies, it is important to realize that adding the expense of a more elaborate and expensive test to a relatively inexpensive one will cost the patient (payor) more than if the more sophisticated procedure had simply been ordered and performed initially.

Because charges vary widely among various institutions and in different geographic regions, the relative costs (technical and professional) listed below are expressed as multiples of the plain frontal and lateral examination of the chest, which is designated as "x".

Barium enema	2.5×
Upper gastrointestinal series	3×
Excretory urogram	3×
Hysterosalpingogram	3×
Ultrasound	3×
Radionuclide scan (lung, bone)	3–4×
Echocardiography	4–5×
CT	7–10×
MRI	8–12×
Angiography	8–12×
CTAP	22×
Surgery	>40×

Index